ACHIEVING GOALS THROUGH STRATEGIC SELF-HYPNOSIS

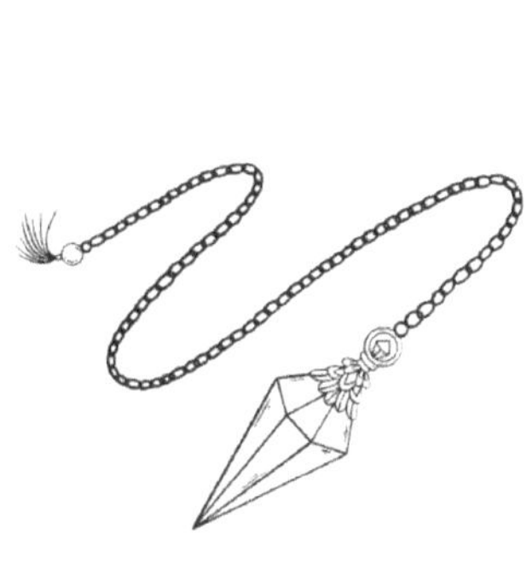 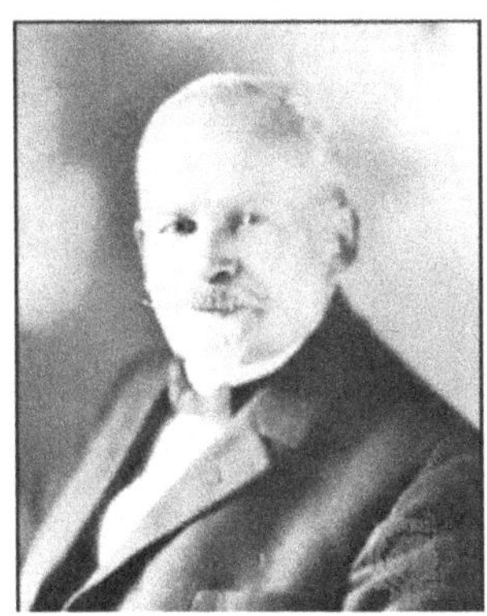

"Hendrina Sterling featuring the principles of Emile Coué's work on self-mastery."

Achieving Goals Through Strategic Self-Hypnosis

By Hendrina Sterling

Counsellor Psychotherapist and Clinical Hypnotherapist

www.MindEmpowerTherapy.com

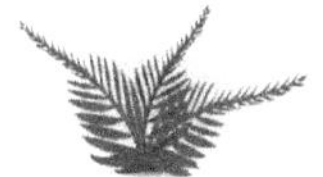

Copyright © 2024 by Hendrina Sterling, United Kingdom.

www.MindEmpowerTherapy.com

Table of Content

Introduction

Coué's philosophy

Émile Coué, a French pharmacist born in 1857, made a big impact in psychology. He believed our thoughts can change our lives. His famous saying, "Every day, in every way, I am getting better and better," shows how repeating positive thoughts can help us.

What's special about Coué is not just his new ideas, but how they show what people can achieve. He thought our subconscious mind, where our hidden thoughts and feelings are, is key to unlocking our abilities. By using auto-suggestion, he said we can tap into this hidden part of our mind and make big changes.

In this read, we'll learn more about Coué's ideas and how they can help us. He had simple ways like saying affirmations over and over, or more complex methods like self-hypnosis, to reach our subconscious. Even though Coué lived over 100 years ago, his ideas still help many people today to overcome challenges and live better lives.

Let's dive into Coué's work with curiosity, ready to discover how our minds can shape our lives through self-belief.

Preface

In the ups and downs of life, there's a powerful tool called self-suggestion. It goes beyond our surface thoughts, diving into our deeper minds where healing and self-control begin.

In this review, we're invited on a journey. It's a journey to break free from suffering and reach our full potential, guided by the wisdom of Professor Coué. His teachings on conscious autosuggestion have helped many find comfort and hope.

Through the stories shared here, we see how self-suggestion can truly change lives. People find relief from pain and escape from despair, showing us the amazing power we each hold inside, just waiting to be tapped into through belief.

This review isn't just stories—it's a guide for those wanting to understand themselves better and grow. For those interested in hypnotherapy or hypnosis, it reveals how our subconscious minds can transform us and teaches techniques to unlock their hidden abilities.

As we read on, let's keep our minds open and our hearts ready to learn. May this review light the way for anyone seeking to navigate life's challenges and discover their true selves.

Warm regards,

Hendrina Sterling

Couéism: The Power of Conscious Autosuggestion

"Tous les jours à tous points de vue je vais de mieux en mieux."

"Every day, in every way, I am getting better and better." (Coué)

At the heart of Émile Coué's philosophy lies the concept of "conscious autosuggestion," a revolutionary method that empowers individuals to harness the latent potential of their own minds. Couéism, as it came to be known, represents a paradigm shift in self-improvement, emphasizing the remarkable influence of suggestion on human behavior and well-being.

"Central to Couéism is the belief that the subconscious mind is receptive to the suggestions it receives, whether positive or negative."

By consciously directing one's thoughts and beliefs, individuals can unlock a reservoir of untapped mental resources, leading to profound personal growth and healing.

Coué's method revolves around the simple yet profound idea that repeated affirmations, spoken with conviction and faith, can shape one's reality. His famous mantra, ***"Every day, in every way, I am getting better and better,"*** encapsulates this principle. Through daily repetition of affirmations, Coué believed that individuals could reprogram their subconscious mind, paving the way for positive change in all aspects of life.

Unlike traditional forms of hypnosis, Couéism does not require the induction of a "trance-like" state. Instead, it emphasizes the power of suggestion in a wakeful, conscious state, making it accessible to anyone willing to practice it diligently.

The key to success in Couéism lies in maintaining a state of relaxed concentration while affirming positive suggestions. By avoiding resistance and embracing a sense of effortlessness, practitioners can bypass the barriers of doubt and skepticism that often impede personal growth.

Coué's legacy continues to inspire countless individuals seeking self-improvement and empowerment. His pioneering work laid the foundation for modern techniques in positive psychology, cognitive-behavioral therapy, and self-help literature.

In essence, Couéism embodies the potential of the human mind and serves as a beacon of hope for those embarking on the journey of self-discovery and personal development. Through the practice of conscious autosuggestion, individuals can unlock their true potential and manifest positive change in their lives.

Autosuggestion

Autosuggestion, as explained before, has been pioneered by Émile Coué at the turn of the 20th century, and it is a psychological technique akin to the placebo effect.

The placebo effect refers to the phenomenon where a person experiences a beneficial effect after receiving a treatment or intervention that has no therapeutic value, simply because they believe it will work. This effect highlights the powerful role of psychological and physiological factors in influencing health outcomes.

Autosuggestion is a process where individuals harness the power of their own thoughts, emotions, and actions through self-induced suggestion. Often employed in self-hypnosis, this technique empowers individuals to shape their mental and emotional states, fostering personal growth and enhancing well-being.

Let's see an example:

"Close your eyes and take a deep breath, allowing yourself to relax completely. With each breath, feel a sense of calmness washing over you. Now, visualize a place where you feel completely at peace, whether it's a serene beach or a quiet forest.

As you immerse yourself in this tranquil scene, repeat positive affirmations to yourself:

'I am calm and centered.'

'I am worthy of love and happiness.'

'I am capable of overcoming any challenge.'

With each affirmation, feel a sense of empowerment growing within you. Imagine these positive thoughts taking root in your mind, replacing any doubts or negativity.

Now, slowly bring your awareness back to the present moment, carrying this sense of peace and positivity with you. Whenever you need a boost, remember these affirmations and the power they hold within you."

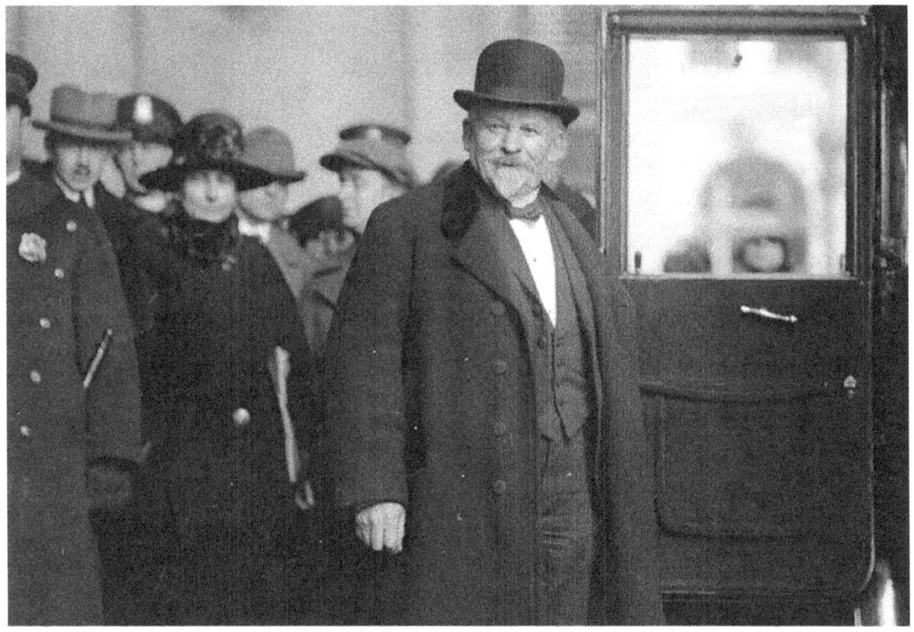

Dr. Emile Coué, 1923 via Wikimedia Commons

Émile Coué made significant contributions to the field of psychology with his development of autosuggestion in the early 20th century. Identifying two distinct types of self-suggestion: *intentional, or "reflective autosuggestion,"* which involves conscious effort, and *unintentional, or "spontaneous auto-suggestion,"* which occurs without conscious intent.

Building upon Coué's insights, his student Charles Baudouin further categorized these suggestions based on their sources: *those stemming from the representative domain, affective domain, and active or motor domain.*

Coué learned about autosuggestion from pharmacology and from top hypnotists like Ambroise-Auguste Liébeault and Hippolyte Bernheim.

Initially drawn to hypnotism, Coué later shifted his focus to autosuggestion, finding inspiration in James Braid's hypnotic techniques. Coué recognized the potential of autosuggestion, particularly in mental therapeutics, and incorporated it into his practice alongside pharmaceutical endeavors. Despite his earlier abandonment of Liébeault's methods, Coué embraced Braid's hypnotism, employing it alongside autosuggestion throughout his career.

Coué's fascination with Bernheim's "suggestive therapeutics" led him to experiment with the power of suggestion in his pharmacy.

"He observed that praising the efficacy of remedies enhanced their effectiveness, a precursor to what we now understand as the placebo response."

One notable instance involved a patent medicine that yielded miraculous cures, despite containing no active ingredients. Coué attributed these results to the patient's continuous self-affirmations, underscoring the potency of autosuggestion in self-healing.

Émile Coué's pioneering work in autosuggestion revolutionized our understanding of the mind's influence on health and well-being. His insights continue to shape modern psychology, highlighting the profound impact of self-suggestion on individual outcomes.

Émile Coué's groundbreaking work led to the birth of "Conscious Autosuggestion," a revolutionary approach to self-improvement and healing. Through his extensive research, Coué discovered that subjects could not be hypnotized against their will and that the effects of hypnotic suggestion faded once subjects regained consciousness. This realization prompted him to develop the Coué method, outlined in his seminal book, ***"Self-Mastery Through Conscious Autosuggestion,"*** first published in England in 1920 and later in the United States.

Coué described autosuggestion as an innate instrument possessed from birth, comparing it to a powerful tool that, when handled consciously, could lead to profound transformations. He emphasized the dual nature of autosuggestion, highlighting its potential to either harm or heal depending on how it was wielded. Coué never dismissed pharmaceutical medicine but rather believed in the synergistic effect of mental state on medication efficacy. He observed that patients who employed his mantra-like suggestion, "Every day, in every way, I'm getting better and better," could enhance the effects of their pharmaceutical treatment by replacing thoughts of illness with thoughts of healing.

It's essential to distinguish Coué's method from other self-administration techniques, such as Autogenic Training developed by Johannes Heinrich

Schultz. While Autogenic Training primarily targets the autonomic nervous system, Coué's approach focuses on saturating the mind with positive suggestions to induce corresponding actions and responses. This conceptual difference underscores the unique effectiveness and versatility of Coué's Conscious Autosuggestion method in promoting holistic well-being and self-improvement.

The Coué method

The Coué method, often misunderstood and reduced to a mere handshake or optimistic mantra, is in fact a sophisticated approach developed through years of careful study, experimentation, and refinement by Émile Coué. Far from being a simplistic technique, it evolved over decades of meticulous observation, theoretical exploration, and practical application.

Its origins can be traced back to around 1901 when Coué initially employed directive hypnotic interventions inspired by techniques learned from an American correspondence course. However, as Coué's understanding of suggestion, autosuggestion, and hypnotism deepened, the method underwent significant transformations.

Gradually, the Coué method evolved into a comprehensive system focused on individual empowerment and self-improvement. It encompassed group education, hypnotherapy, ego-strengthening exercises, and training in self-suggested pain control. Central to the method was the unique formula repeated twice daily by practitioners:

"Every day, in every way, I'm getting better and better."

This final iteration of the Coué method emphasized the intentional and deliberate application of autosuggestion, empowering individuals to take control of their mental and physical well-being. Through Coué's method, countless individuals have discovered the power of positive self-talk and self-directed change.

The Coué method revolves around the repetitive use of a specific expression, following a prescribed ritual, in a particular physical state, and without the inclusion of any associated mental imagery, both at the beginning and end of each day. Coué believed that effecting change in our subconscious or unconscious thoughts, which can only be achieved through the use of our imagination, is crucial for overcoming certain troubles. While he emphasized that he was not primarily a healer but rather a teacher guiding others to heal themselves, Coué asserted that he could induce organic changes through autosuggestion.

Central to Coué's method are several underlying principles:

"He suggested that any idea frequently on the mind can become real, as long as it's possible."

For instance, while someone without hands cannot regrow them, a person firmly believing their asthma is disappearing may experience improvement to the extent that the body can physically overcome or manage the illness. Conversely, negative thoughts about illness can reinforce its presence.

Coué identified willpower as a primary obstacle to successful autosuggestion. Patients must refrain from imposing their willpower and judgments on positive ideas for the method to be effective. Coué observed that young children often applied his method flawlessly due to their lack of strong willpower compared to adults.

He also warned against self-conflict, where willpower and imagination oppose each other, leading to exacerbated problems. To achieve success, patients must relinquish willpower and focus on harnessing their imaginative power.

The effectiveness of Coué's method is evidenced by numerous case studies where patients experienced improvements in various physical and mental ailments. However, advocates of autosuggestion acknowledge the need for further scientific evidence to substantiate its efficacy.

Autogenic training, influenced by the Coué method, is a relaxation technique developed by German psychiatrist Johannes Schultz in 1932. Unlike autosuggestion, autogenic training has been validated in clinical trials and is administered by qualified professionals. Its effectiveness has been demonstrated in numerous studies, making it a widely accepted therapeutic approach.

While the Coué method laid the groundwork for understanding the power of autosuggestion, autogenic training has emerged as a more scientifically validated relaxation technique in therapy.

Refinement of Autosuggestion Techniques: General and Specific Approaches

1. The General Method:

"Every day, in every way, I am getting better and better." This foundational mantra, recited at least 20 times each evening in a tranquil, whispered cadence, serves as a gateway to profound self-improvement. Coué advises employing closed-eyed introspection, accompanied by the gentle counting of rosary beads, reminiscent of ancient mantra practices. However, he wisely cautions against excessive fixation, urging practitioners to imbue the phrase with personal significance. Central to its effectiveness is the deliberate reflection on individual therapeutic objectives, fostering a deep connection with the affirmation's meaning. Coué further advocates periodic reaffirmation during brief intervals of self-hypnosis throughout the day, reinforcing the subconscious directive for holistic enhancement.

2. The Specific Method:

For targeted relief from acute distress or pain, Coué prescribes the succinct phrase, "It is going," or in French, "ça passe." Rapid, almost hurried repetition is key, preventing the intrusion of conflicting thoughts and facilitating swift absorption by the subconscious mind. Coué recommends light, repetitive gestures—gentle rubs over afflicted areas or soothing strokes across the forehead—to synchronize physical action with verbal affirmation. In his instructional sessions, he exemplifies this technique, encouraging participants to emulate the rhythmic recitation and accompanying movements. Persistence is paramount, with Coué advocating relentless application until discomfort subsides. He underscores the virtue of patience, assuring that sustained practice will diminish reliance on the method over time. Baudouin, echoing Coué's wisdom, emphasizes the balance between swift recitation for sensory-focused suggestions and measured delivery for deeper, introspective directives. While cautioning against unnecessary complexity, he extols the accessibility and efficacy of Coué's approach, urging practitioners to trust in its simplicity.

Émile Coué's ideas gained traction primarily through his seminars and word-of-mouth recommendations. He possessed a unique charisma that left a lasting impression on those who encountered him. Charles Baudouin, in a preface to his book, vividly described Coué's character, portraying him as unpretentious and ever-ready to lend a helping hand. A photograph capturing Coué surrounded by a large group of patients further attests to the popularity of his free-of-charge group clinics, held in Troyes and later in Nancy.

According to Baudouin, Coué treated a staggering number of patients each day, conducting thousands of consultations annually. His approach was characterized by a direct and sometimes forceful manner of speaking, often using simple English with a distinct Gallic accent and temperament. While some have dubbed him the father of modern "self-help," it's important to note that self-help literature predates his time.

The enduring popularity of Coué's methods is evident in the widespread recognition of "Couéism." This phenomenon is perhaps best illustrated by the inclusion of a description of the Coué method in the lyrics of the well-known pop song "Beautiful Boy" by John Lennon.

"Beautiful, beautiful, beautiful, beautiful boy,

"Before you go to sleep,

"Say a little prayer,

"Every day in every way,

"It's getting better and better."

- John Lennon, Beautiful Boy (Darling Boy), 1980

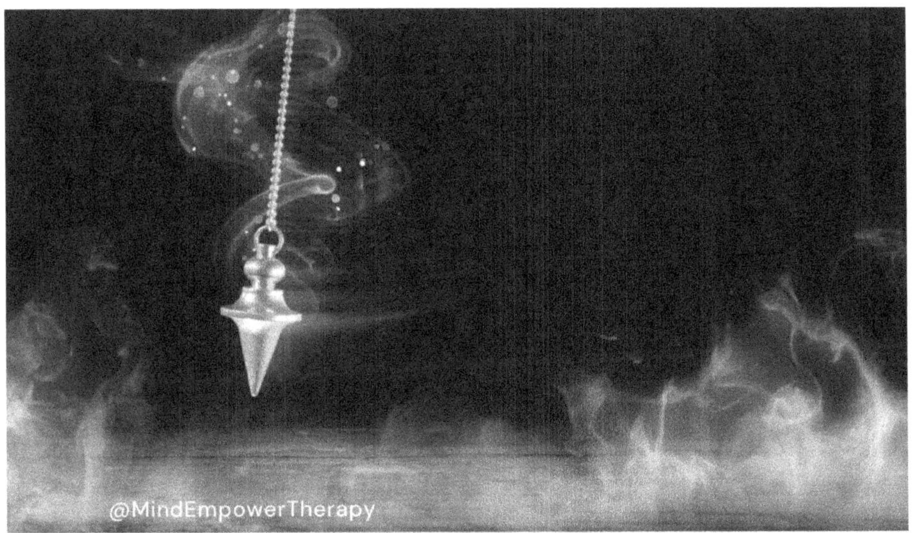

The Laws of Autosuggestion

The Laws of Autosuggestion, foundational to Couéism, are rooted in two fundamental theoretical principles:

"All suggestion is autosuggestion."

"Internal conflict arises between the will and imagination, with the imagination prevailing in strength." (q.v., Coué, 1923: 19).

These principles lay the groundwork for understanding the dynamics of autosuggestion and its impact on individual behavior and outcomes.

The Law of Concentrated Attention

The first law, the Law of Concentrated Attention, posits that ideas upon which attention is concentrated are amplified in their influence. Spontaneous autosuggestions can naturally seize attention, while conscious autosuggestions require deliberate repetition with mental focus, certainty, and faith. This principle mirrors Braid's concept of hypnotism as the focused concentration on a dominant idea, known as "monoideism."

The Law of Auxiliary Emotion

The second law, the Law of Auxiliary Emotion, suggests that when an idea is imbued with strong emotion, it is more likely to be realized suggestively.

Emotion plays an auxiliary role in capturing attention and translating an idea into action, particularly evident in spontaneous negative autosuggestion. Negative ideas persist in our minds due to the potent emotions, notably fear, attached to them. This emotional intensity gives spontaneous autosuggestion an initial advantage over deliberate conscious autosuggestion, as the latter often lacks such strong and genuine emotion.

The Law of Reversed Effort

The third law, the Law of Reversed Effort, presents a challenge to the use of autosuggestion by highlighting that the more one consciously struggles against a dominant idea, the more powerful its effects become. Efforts to counteract a suggestion actually reinforce it, as conscious attempts to resist intensify the suggestion. This is demonstrated by the self-defeating mindset of "I would like to... but I cannot." This concept bears resemblance to modern reverse psychology, a persuasion technique that aims to persuade by suggesting the opposite.

To overcome this obstacle, the New Nancy School recommended using conscious autosuggestion effortlessly, without tension or excessive effort. Suggestions should be made naturally, simply, and with conviction, without striving through willpower. It emphasizes imagining things as easy and already on the path to accomplishment, rather than struggling with them forcefully.

The Law of Subconscious Teleology

The fourth law, the Law of Subconscious Teleology, asserts that once an end or goal has been suggested, the subconscious mind will find ways to realize it. Autosuggestion directs attention towards the desired outcome, allowing the subconscious to spontaneously devise means for its attainment. While this approach is generally conducive to autosuggestion, it is important to note that for complex or long-term goals, breaking them down into manageable steps and stages is often advisable. This is because the mind may have limitations in spontaneously working out solutions for such goals.

The Law of Inverted Effort

Émile Coué illuminates a fundamental truth: the exertion of willpower against the current of imagination merely amplifies its force. He astutely observes that endeavors to suppress phenomena like stage fright or nervous laughter often intensify them. According to Coué's doctrine, when negative ideas dominate the psyche, futile resistance only serves to reinforce them, plunging the individual deeper into the quicksand of their own negativity.

For Coué and his adherents, the Law of Inverted Effort stands as the cornerstone of his revolutionary method. Vigorous attempts at conscious control, bereft of positive counter-ideas, inadvertently bolster the undesirable mental image. Coué poignantly likens this struggle to a futile battle against sinking in quicksand—a metaphor for the neurotic's futile attempts to resist negative autosuggestions.

Baudouin, an ardent proponent of Coué's philosophy, underscores the centrality of this law. He warns against excessive effort, which only serves to evoke antagonistic thoughts, leading to counterproductive ideo-reflex responses. In this state of cognitive dissonance, conflicting suggestions neutralize each other, often yielding negative outcomes. Coué himself champions the belief in effortless change, stressing that challenges are only as formidable as one perceives them to be. Effortlessness, he asserts, is a habit to be cultivated, essential for the practice of autosuggestion.

Despite the paradox of urging effortlessness while engaging the imagination, Coué advocates the channeling of willpower solely for the initial direction of the imagination. He advises practicing autosuggestion during periods of drowsiness, when conscious effort naturally wanes. Rapid repetition during waking hours prevents the intrusion of antagonistic thoughts, aligning with Coué's principle of effortless suggestion.

Indeed, Coué's insights into the laws of suggestion find resonance in scientific experiments like Chevreul's pendulum, where attempts to halt motion through sheer willpower often yield the opposite effect, reinforcing the wisdom of surrendering to the flow of imagination.

The Nancy School

The Nancy School, rooted in the pioneering work of Ambroise-Auguste Liébeault in 1866, emerged as a leading French hypnosis-centered psychotherapy school in Nancy, France. Liébeault's influential publications and therapy sessions attracted attention, notably from Dr. Hippolyte Bernheim, also based in Nancy. Bernheim played a crucial role in refining Liébeault's ideas, leading to the establishment of the Nancy School.

Unlike the Paris School, which focused on hysteria-centered hypnosis research led by Jean-Martin Charcot in Paris, the Nancy School took a different approach. While the Paris School emphasized dramatic hysteria manifestations under hypnosis, the Nancy School prioritized a collaborative and suggestive therapy approach, highlighting the power of suggestion in achieving therapeutic results.

The contributions of the Nancy School laid the groundwork for modern hypnosis and psychotherapy, influencing the development of therapeutic techniques and methodologies still used today. Its impact is evident in widespread acceptance and application, with numerous studies demonstrating the safety and effectiveness of Nancy School techniques in various contexts.

Clinical evidence highlights the therapeutic benefits of Nancy School techniques, particularly in managing pain and anxiety, and potentially addressing conditions like dementia. The versatility of hypnosis and suggestion is seen in their ability to address a range of issues, from smoking cessation to headache management.

The influence of the Nancy School extends beyond psychology, shaping the work of prominent figures in the field such as Morton Prince and Auguste Forel. Even Freud, often seen as the father of psychoanalysis, was influenced by Nancy School principles, incorporating hypnotism into his therapeutic approach.

Émile Coué furthered the Nancy School's legacy with his Coué Method, demonstrating its ongoing relevance and evolution in addressing modern challenges.

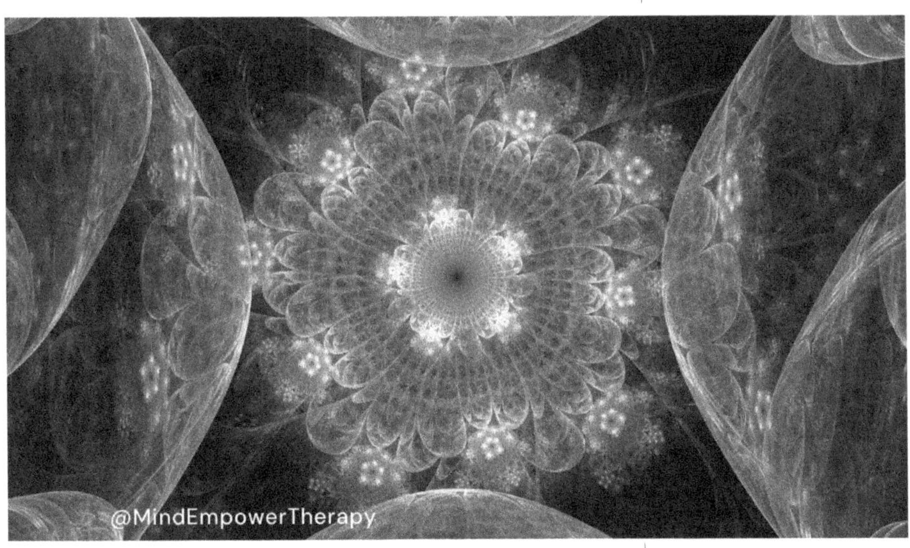

Self-hypnosis

James Braid, a Scottish physician and surgeon, is credited with introducing the term *"hypnotism"* in 1841. Braid's interest in hypnotism led him to experiment with what he termed *"self-hypnotism"* or self-hypnosis, which he first practiced in 1843. He recounted his experiences with self-hypnosis in his work **"Observations on Trance or Human Hybernation"** published in 1850.

In this work, Braid described a severe bout of rheumatism he experienced in September 1844, which left him in excruciating pain, deprived of sleep for three nights. Despite trying various medications without relief, he decided to try self-hypnosis as a last resort. With the assistance of two friends who were knowledgeable about hypnotism, Braid induced a hypnotic state in himself and found that, to his surprise, the pain completely disappeared. He continued to practice self-hypnosis whenever he experienced a recurrence of the rheumatism, ultimately remaining free from the condition for nearly six years.

Braid's personal experience with self-hypnosis provided him with firsthand evidence of its effectiveness in managing pain and promoting healing. His pioneering work laid the foundation for further exploration and understanding of hypnotism as a therapeutic tool.

Self-hypnosis, also known as auto-hypnosis, involves inducing a hypnotic state in oneself through various techniques. Unlike hetero-hypnosis, where one person hypnotizes another, self-hypnosis is a process where the individual plays both the role of the suggester and the suggestee.

In self-hypnosis, individuals often utilize the hypnotic state to enhance the effectiveness of self-suggestion. This dual role allows them to suggest positive changes or outcomes to themselves, harnessing the power of their subconscious mind.

The practice of self-hypnosis can vary in focus and approach. In concentrative self-hypnosis, individuals maintain intense focus on a specific suggestion or mantra, such as "Every day, in every way, I'm getting better and better," excluding all other thoughts and distractions from their awareness. On the other hand, inclusive self-hypnosis involves allowing various thoughts, emotions, memories, and sensations to enter consciousness while still maintaining a hypnotic state.

Overall, self-hypnosis serves as a tool for individuals to access their subconscious mind and enact positive changes through self-suggestion. By mastering this technique, individuals can empower themselves to overcome obstacles, achieve goals, and enhance their overall well-being.

Émile Coué played a significant role in the development of self-hypnosis. His method of "conscious autosuggestion" gained widespread recognition as a powerful self-help system in the early 20th century. Although Coué preferred to distance himself from the term "hypnosis," he occasionally referred to his technique as self-hypnosis, a perspective shared by his followers like Charles Baudouin. Today, modern hypnotherapists consider Coué's contributions to be integral to their field.

Another notable relaxation technique, **'autogenic training'**, was developed by German psychiatrist Johannes Schultz and first published in

1932. Schultz drew inspiration from the work of German hypnotist Oskar Vogt. Autogenic training follows a structured progression, starting with physiological conditioning such as muscle relaxation, breathing control, and heart rate regulation. It then advances to psychic conditioning through techniques like mental imagery and acoustic therapy.

These are the steps commonly used for self-hypnosis:

Motivation: Because having a strong motivation is essential for effective self-hypnosis practice. Without proper motivation, it can be challenging to focus and achieve desired outcomes.

Relaxation: The individual must achieve a deep state of relaxation, free from distractions. This often involves setting aside dedicated time and creating a calm environment conducive to relaxation.

Concentration: Complete concentration is necessary during self-hypnosis. Focusing the mind on a single image or thought helps to induce a hypnotic state and deepen the experience.

Directing: This step involves directing one's concentration toward a specific goal or desired outcome. By visualizing the desired result during the hypnotic state, individuals can work on achieving their objectives effectively.

Uses of self-hypnosis:

- **Pain management:** Self-hypnosis has been effective in alleviating physical pain, reducing tension, and promoting relaxation.
- **Anxiety and stress reduction:** It can help individuals manage anxiety, reduce stress levels, and promote overall emotional well-being.

- **Depression:** Self-hypnosis techniques may aid in managing symptoms of depression and improving mood.
- **Sleep disorders:** It can be used to promote better sleep quality and address insomnia.
- **Weight loss:** Self-hypnosis can support weight loss efforts by influencing behaviors, attitudes, and motivations related to food and exercise.
- **Asthma and skin conditions:** It has shown potential in managing asthma symptoms and improving skin conditions through relaxation and stress reduction.
- **Enhancing cognitive abilities:** Self-hypnosis can improve concentration, memory recall, problem-solving skills, and emotional control.
- **Childbirth anesthesia:** Women in labor can use self-hypnosis techniques to manage pain and anxiety during childbirth, with methods such as glove anesthesia, time distortion, and imaginative transformation.

Overall, self-hypnosis offers a versatile approach to address various issues and behavioral challenges, empowering individuals to take control of their mental and physical well-being through self-directed thought and suggestion.

"When it comes to autosuggestion, Coué emphasizes..."

"It is a sort of little trick. When one learns the trick he is able to become master of himself." (Coué, 1923: 119)

Mastering Yourself Through Mindful Self-Suggestion

But where the concept of suggestion comes from? This concept or more specifically autosuggestion, is relatively contemporary, yet it's as ancient as human existence itself. Its novelty lies in the fact that it has often been misinterpreted and misunderstood until now. However, its antiquity traces back to the dawn of humanity.

"Autosuggestion is an inherent tool we possess from birth, harboring within it an incredible and immeasurable power that can yield both positive and negative outcomes depending on the circumstances."

Understanding this power is beneficial to everyone, but it holds particular significance for professionals such as doctors, judges, lawyers, and educators. By mastering conscious practice of autosuggestion, we can firstly prevent inadvertently inducing harmful suggestions in others, which could lead to disastrous outcomes. Secondly, we can intentionally stimulate positive suggestions, thereby promoting physical well-being for the sick and psychological well-being for those suffering from neurosis or misguided behavior – individuals who are often victims of subconscious suggestions from their past. Additionally, we can help steer individuals with a predisposition towards making wrong choices onto the right path."

The Conscious Self and the Unconscious Self

This is an important point. To grasp the intricacies of suggestion, or more accurately, autosuggestion, it's essential to recognize the existence of two distinct selves within us: ***"the conscious and the unconscious."*** While both possess intelligence, the conscious self is aware, while the unconscious remains hidden, often escaping notice. However, its presence becomes evident upon closer examination of certain phenomena such as behaviour and life's issues.

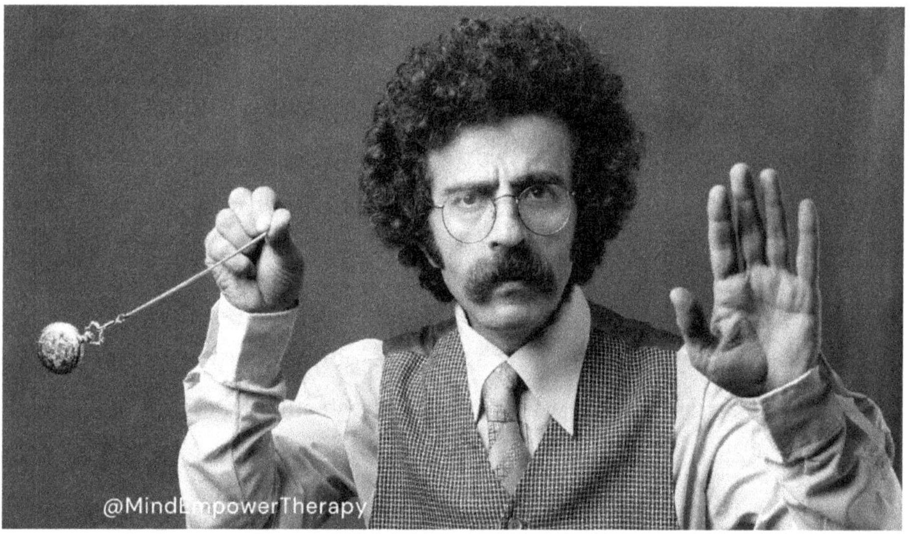

Consider somnambulism, a phenomenon familiar to many. A somnambulist arises from slumber without awakening, engages in various activities, and then returns to bed, often unaware of their actions. Who or what guides these actions if not an unconscious force—the individual's unconscious self?

Similarly, consider the unfortunate scenario of a drunkard experiencing delirium tremens. In a frenzy, they may wield nearby objects as weapons, causing harm without awareness. Afterward, they may be horrified by the aftermath, oblivious to their own actions. Once again, it is the unconscious self that drives such behavior.

In comparing the conscious and unconscious selves, we observe that the conscious self often possesses an unreliable memory, whereas the unconscious self boasts a remarkable and flawless memory, recording even the minutest details of our existence. Moreover, the unconscious self is credulous, readily accepting information without skepticism.

Remarkably, the unconscious self governs not only bodily functions but also all actions, including those driven by imagination. Despite common belief, it is the unconscious self that compels us to act, sometimes against our conscious will, particularly when there is conflict between these two forces. Thus, understanding and harnessing the power of conscious autosuggestions against negative unconscious influences can lead to the alleviation of unjust suffering and the realization of positive outcomes.

Will and Imagination

When we consult a dictionary for the definition of "will," we encounter the notion of "the faculty of freely determining certain acts." This definition, however, is far from accurate. Contrary to popular belief, our will invariably succumbs to the power of imagination. It's an unyielding truth with no exceptions.

You might initially balk at this assertion, dismissing it as blasphemy or paradox. But upon closer examination, you'll find it to be the purest truth, not a fanciful theory concocted by a troubled mind.

Consider this: envision a plank, 30 feet long and 1 foot wide, lying flat on the ground. It's evident that anyone could walk across it without fear of falling off. Now, alter the scenario. Imagine the same plank suspended high above the ground, between the towers of a cathedral. Who among us would dare to venture even a few steps along this precarious path? The mere thought of it induces trembling, regardless of our willpower. Despite our best intentions, we'd likely succumb to the ground below.

Why does this happen? Because our ability to advance is not governed by our will alone. It's dictated by our imagination. When the plank lies on the ground, we believe it's easy to traverse. But when it's elevated, we convince ourselves it's impossible.

Consider vertigo—a sensation entirely conjured by the mental image of falling. Despite our efforts to resist, this image materializes into reality, thwarting our intentions.

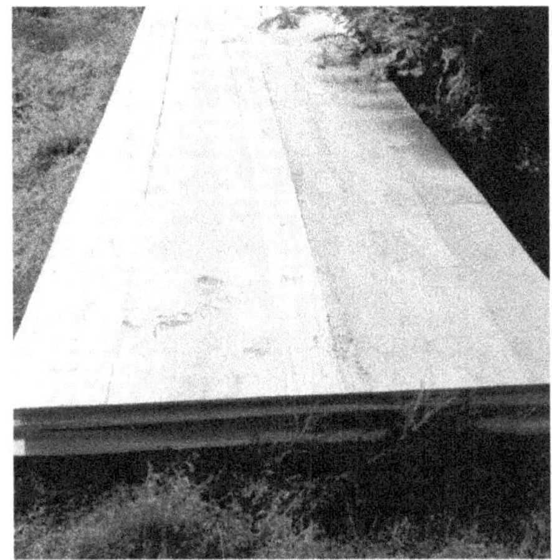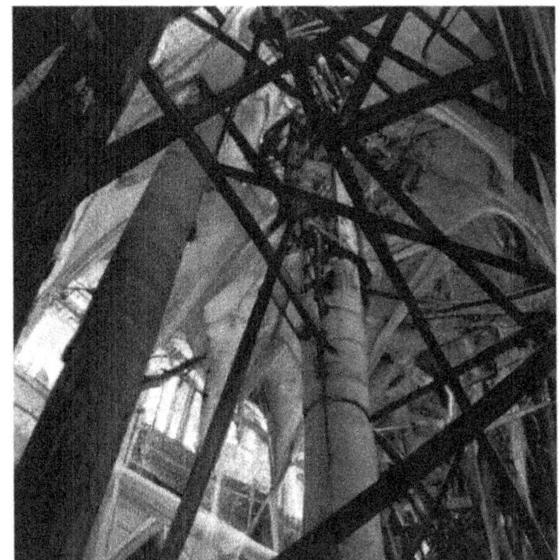

Similarly, imagine struggling with insomnia. The more we will ourselves to sleep, the more elusive it becomes. It's a paradoxical dance: the harder we try, the further sleep slips away.

Think also of the frustration of forgetting someone's name. The more we strain to recall it, the more it evades us. Yet, when we relinquish our efforts and simply trust that the name will return, it does so effortlessly.

In essence, our will is no match for the power of imagination. It's a humbling realization that underscores the profound influence of our thoughts on our actions and experiences.

Reflect on your experiences as a cyclist learning to ride. Gripping the handlebars tightly, you feared falling and anxiously avoided even the smallest obstacles, only to find yourself drawn toward them with greater force the harder you tried to evade them.

Think also of uncontrollable laughter—an eruption that intensifies despite your efforts to suppress it.

In each of these scenarios, examine the inner conflict: "I don't want to fall, but I can't prevent it"; "I want to sleep, but I'm unable to"; "I want to remember a name, but it eludes me"; "I want to avoid the obstacle, but I can't"; "I want to stop laughing, but I can't."

Notice how, without exception, the imagination triumphs over the will.

Consider the leader who galvanizes their troops forward, inspiring unity and momentum. Conversely, the cry of "Every man for himself!" often leads to defeat. Why? Because in the former, soldiers imagine pressing onward, while in the latter, they imagine defeat and flight.

Reflect on Panurge's shrewd manipulation of imagination, as he orchestrated the actions of his fellow passengers by tossing a sheep overboard, knowing the rest would follow suit.

Humans, like sheep, are prone to following others' examples, driven by an irresistible impulse rooted in imagination.

Consider those battling addiction, sincerely desiring sobriety yet feeling compelled to drink against their will. Similarly, certain criminals commit acts they abhor, feeling powerless to resist the impulses driving them.

These examples underscore the immense power of imagination—or, in other words, the unconscious—in its struggle against the will.

Indeed, some drinkers and criminals are truthful when they claim they cannot control their actions; they are shackled by the belief that they lack agency.

Despite our pride in our willpower and freedom, we often find ourselves at the mercy of our imagination, mere puppets with our imagination pulling the strings. Only when we learn to harness and direct our imagination do we transcend our puppet-like existence.

Suggestion and Autosuggestion

Regarding suggestion and autosuggestion, Emile Coué employs vivid analogies to illustrate the dynamic between the imagination and the unconscious mind, emphasizing their potential for both chaos and control.

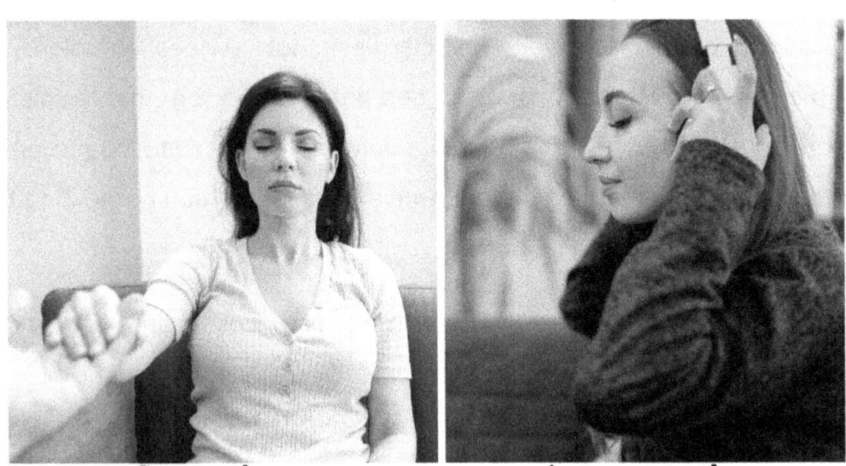

Coué likens the imagination to a torrent, a powerful force that can overwhelm an individual despite their efforts to resist. However, he suggests that with the right approach, this torrent can be redirected and harnessed for productive purposes, much like channeling its force into a factory to generate movement, heat, and electricity.

Alternatively, Coué paints a picture of the imagination as an unbridled horse, capable of running wild and leading its rider astray. Without proper guidance, the rider is at the mercy of the horse's whims, often ending up in a metaphorical ditch. Yet, when the rider succeeds in imposing control by fitting the horse with a bridle, the balance of power shifts, and the rider dictates the direction of their journey.

Having established the formidable nature of the unconscious or imaginative self, Coué sets out to demonstrate how it can be tamed and directed. However, before delving into practical methods, he emphasizes the importance of understanding two fundamental concepts: suggestion and autosuggestion.

Suggestion, Coué explains, involves imposing an idea onto another individual's brain. However, he clarifies that suggestion alone is insufficient; it must be absorbed and internalized by the recipient's unconscious mind to become effective autosuggestion. Autosuggestion, in contrast, entails implanting an idea within oneself, thereby harnessing the power of one's own unconscious.

Coué illustrates the concept by recounting instances where suggestions failed to yield results because the subject's unconscious mind did not accept and transform them into autosuggestions. This underscores the critical role of the unconscious in the process of suggestion and the importance of aligning conscious intentions with unconscious acceptance.

In essence, Coué lays the groundwork for understanding how suggestion and autosuggestion operate in tandem to influence behavior and shape outcomes. He sets the stage for exploring practical techniques to leverage autosuggestion effectively in achieving personal transformation and self-mastery.

Suggestion and autosuggestion, as previously discussed, can be likened to the untamed force of a torrent or an unbridled horse. They possess immense power, sweeping individuals away or leading them on reckless paths unless properly directed.

Consider suggestion as the act of implanting an idea onto another's mind. However, suggestion alone does not hold sway unless it transforms into autosuggestion within the individual. Autosuggestion, on the other hand, is the process of implanting an idea within oneself.

You may offer a suggestion to someone, but if their unconscious mind does not accept and internalize it, transforming it into autosuggestion, it remains ineffectual. Even obedient subjects may reject suggestions if their unconscious minds refuse to digest and convert them into autosuggestions.

I've encountered situations where I made seemingly straightforward suggestions to highly compliant individuals, only to witness their lack of success. This occurred because their unconscious minds rejected the suggestions, failing to transform them into autosuggestions.

Expanding upon the analogy of the imagination as a torrent or an unbridled horse, we can delve deeper into the transformative power of suggestion and autosuggestion.

Imagine the imagination as a wild torrent, capable of sweeping individuals away in its tumultuous current. Despite their efforts to resist, they find themselves powerless against its force. However, with knowledge and skill, one can redirect this torrent, guiding it towards productive ends. Just as a skilled engineer can divert a river's flow to power a factory, we can harness the energy of our imagination, converting it into action, creativity, and innovation.

Alternatively, consider the imagination as an untamed horse, lacking bridle and reins. Without control, it gallops recklessly, dragging its rider along unpredictable paths. Yet, with the proper tools and techniques, the rider can assert dominance, guiding the horse with precision and purpose. In this way, the rider becomes the master, dictating the direction and pace of their journey.

Having recognized the formidable power of the unconscious or imaginative mind, we can explore how to exert control over it. It's akin to taming the torrent or breaking in the wild horse. But before delving into these techniques, it's essential to clarify the concepts of suggestion and autosuggestion.

Suggestion, defined as the act of implanting an idea onto another's mind, relies on the subsequent transformation into autosuggestion within the individual. Autosuggestion, in turn, is the process of internalizing an idea within oneself, shaping beliefs and behaviors accordingly.

Consider this: you may offer a suggestion to someone, but its effectiveness hinges on their unconscious acceptance and transformation into autosuggestion. Even among typically compliant individuals, suggestions may fail to take root if their unconscious minds resist or reject them.

I've encountered instances where seemingly straightforward suggestions proved ineffective, as the subject's unconscious mind refused to internalize them. This highlights the importance of understanding and harnessing the power of autosuggestion—a skill that empowers individuals to shape their thoughts, beliefs, and actions consciously. Through mastering autosuggestion, we can effectively guide our imagination, transforming its energy into productive endeavors and fulfilling achievements.

The Suggestion Effect Experiment: An Illustration of the Power of Will and Imagination

Let's delve into an experiential exercise to vividly grasp the principles advocated by Coué. Begin by standing on your feet, observing your hands. With deliberate intent, bring your hands together as if preparing to clap. Then, slowly allow your hands to part, focusing intently on the movement. Repeat this sequence three times, maintaining your focus on the action of opening your hands and arms.

Now, as your hands remain open, take a moment to try closing them slowly. You may notice a subtle resistance or a sensation akin to an invisible force preventing your hands from reuniting. What could be the underlying force that seems to keep your hands from coming together? Explore this intriguing question as we unravel the dynamics of willpower and imagination."

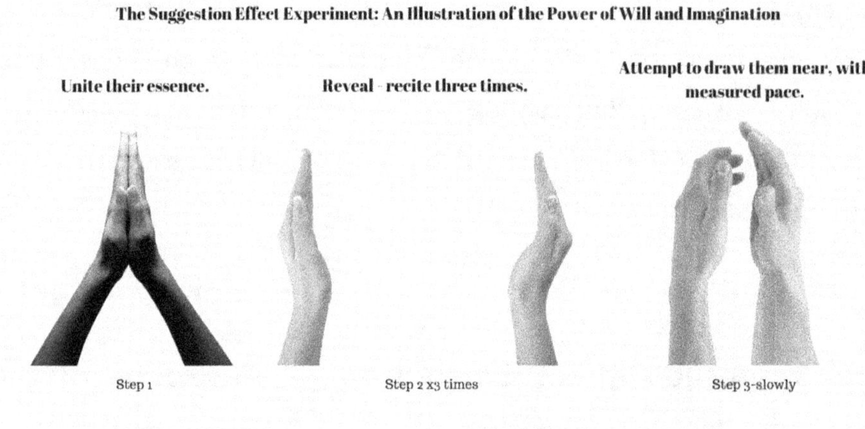

The Use of Autosuggestion

In ***"The Use of Autosuggestion,"*** Emile Coué reveals the transformative power of harnessing one's imagination through conscious autosuggestion, offering a practical guide to unlocking its potential for personal growth and healing.

Coué likens the unconscious mind to a powerful force, comparable to a torrent or an untamed horse, capable of leading individuals astray if left unchecked. However, he asserts that with awareness and guidance, this force can be directed towards positive outcomes, much like redirecting a torrent's flow to power a factory or fitting a bridle on a horse to control its path.

It involves consciously implanting ideas within oneself, thereby influencing both mental and physical well-being. By repetitively affirming positive statements, individuals can prompt their unconscious to accept and act upon these suggestions, leading to tangible results.

Coué emphasizes the simplicity of autosuggestion, noting that it is a natural ability inherent in all individuals from birth. However, he warns of its potential dangers when wielded unconsciously, likening it to a double-edged sword that can either harm or heal depending on how it is used.

To illustrate the power of conscious autosuggestion, Coué provides examples of individuals who have successfully overcome various challenges by changing their internal dialogue. He highlights the role of imagination in shaping reality, demonstrating how beliefs and expectations can influence outcomes.

Furthermore, Coué dispels common misconceptions about willpower, asserting that imagination invariably triumphs over will in shaping behavior. He outlines fundamental principles governing the interplay between will and imagination, underscoring the importance of aligning conscious intentions with unconscious acceptance.

Despite the potential of autosuggestion to facilitate healing and personal development, Coué acknowledges that some individuals may struggle to embrace it fully. He identifies two groups—those mentally undeveloped and those unwilling to understand—as less receptive to conscious autosuggestion, emphasizing the need for patience and persistence in guiding them towards its benefits.

In essence, Coué's exploration of autosuggestion offers a roadmap for individuals to tap into their inner resources and cultivate a positive mindset. By harnessing the power of imagination through conscious autosuggestion, individuals can transcend limitations, overcome challenges, and lead more fulfilling lives.

Emile Coué provides to illustrate the power of conscious autosuggestion:

- ***Overcoming Neurasthenia:*** Coué discusses individuals who believe themselves incapable of exerting even the slightest effort due to neurasthenia. He explains how their belief in their limitations leads to exhaustion, creating a self-perpetuating cycle of physical and mental fatigue.
- ***Managing Pain:*** Coué demonstrates how one's perception of pain can be altered through autosuggestion. By convincing oneself that a pain is diminishing, individuals can actually experience relief as their unconscious mind accepts and acts upon this suggestion.
- ***Predicting Illness:*** He mentions individuals who anticipate and even induce sickness through autosuggestion. By convincing themselves that they will experience a headache or other ailment on a particular day, in specific circumstances, they manifest these symptoms as a result of their own beliefs.
- ***Psychological Paralysis:*** Coué discusses cases where individuals become paralyzed without any physical cause, attributing their condition to unconscious autosuggestion. Through the power of imagination, they convince themselves of their paralysis, leading to tangible physical effects.

- ***Emotional States:*** He highlights the role of autosuggestion in shaping emotional states, suggesting that individuals can make themselves happy or unhappy by imagining themselves as such. This demonstrates the profound influence of belief systems on one's subjective experience of reality.

These examples showcase the breadth of applications for conscious autosuggestion, ranging from physical healing to emotional well-being. They underscore Coué's central premise that the mind possesses the inherent capacity to influence and shape one's reality through deliberate and focused thought patterns.

Let's revisit the concept that we can control and direct our imagination, much like one can manage a torrent or tame an unbroken horse. Achieving this requires two key realizations: first, understanding that this control is possible (a fact often overlooked by many), and second, knowing the method by which it can be achieved. This method is remarkably simple—it's something we've been doing unconsciously since birth, though often incorrectly and to our detriment. This method is autosuggestion.

While we continually give ourselves unconscious autosuggestions, the key lies in giving ourselves conscious ones. Here's how it works: carefully consider the desired outcome in your mind, and then repeat to yourself several times, without distraction: "This thing is coming," or "this thing is going away"; "this thing will happen," or "this thing will not happen," and so forth. If the unconscious mind accepts and transforms this suggestion into autosuggestion, the desired outcome becomes a reality in every aspect.

Of course, it's essential to note that the thing being suggested must be within our control.

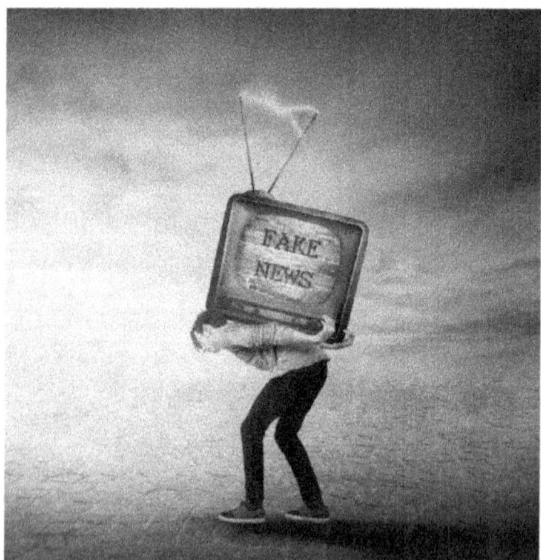
Suggestion

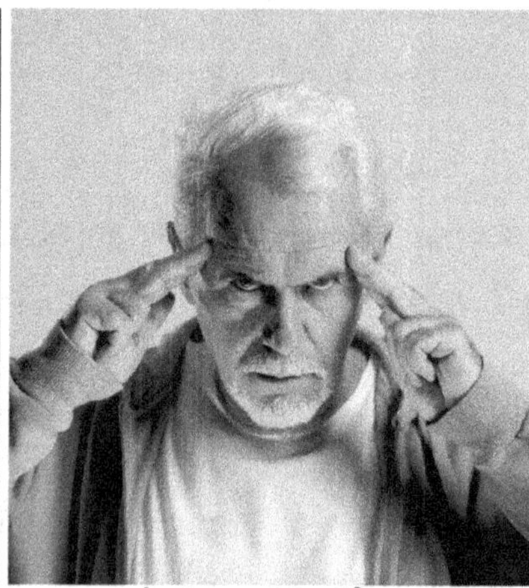
Autosuggestion

In essence, autosuggestion can be understood as a form of self-hypnosis. It's the influence of the imagination on both the mental and physical aspects of our being. This influence is undeniable, and I'll refrain from revisiting previous examples, opting instead to provide a few additional illustrations.

The power of belief cannot be overstated. If you convince yourself that you can accomplish a task, as long as it's within the realm of possibility, you will find a way to do it, no matter how daunting it may seem. Conversely, if you convince yourself that even the simplest of tasks is beyond your capability, you will indeed find it impossible to accomplish, turning minor obstacles into insurmountable barriers.

Consider individuals suffering from neurasthenia. Believing themselves incapable of exertion, they often struggle to even take a few steps without feeling utterly drained. Their condition worsens the more they try to fight it, akin to a person sinking deeper into quicksand the more they struggle.

Similarly, the power of suggestion is evident in the realm of pain management. Merely believing that a pain is fading can lead to its gradual disappearance, while believing that one is experiencing pain can trigger its onset.

I've observed individuals who predict the onset of a headache on a particular day under specific circumstances, and predictably, they experience it as expected. Their belief in their impending illness becomes a self-fulfilling prophecy, just as others are able to cure themselves through conscious autosuggestion.

It may sound unconventional, but I firmly believe that many mental and physical ailments stem from unconscious autosuggestion—the influence of the unconscious mind on our physical and mental well-being. Neurasthenia, stammering, aversions, kleptomania, and even certain cases of paralysis can be traced back to this phenomenon.

However, just as our unconscious mind can be the source of our ailments, it also possesses the power to heal. Its influence on our organism is profound, capable not only of repairing the harm it has caused but also of curing genuine illnesses. This underscores the remarkable potential of our unconscious mind to shape our health and well-being in profound ways.

Harness the power of autosuggestion

To harness the power of autosuggestion, find a quiet space, sit comfortably in an armchair, and close your eyes to eliminate distractions. Focus your mind on a specific thought: **"Such and such a thing is going to disappear,"** or **"Such and such a thing is coming to pass."**

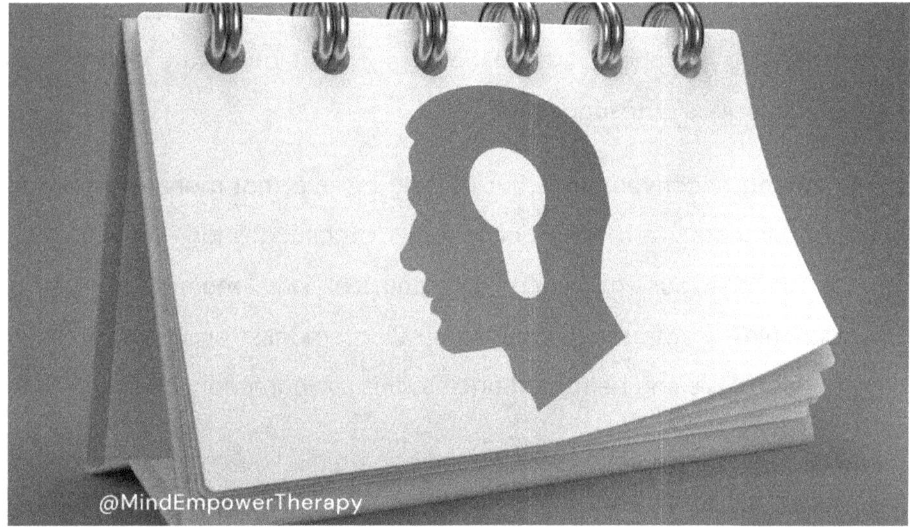

As you engage in this mental exercise, it's crucial to note that the effectiveness of autosuggestion hinges on whether your unconscious mind has truly absorbed the idea you've presented to it. You may be surprised to witness the realization of the thought you've focused on. It's important to recognize that ideas suggested to our unconscious often exist within us unnoticed, only revealing themselves through the effects they produce.

An essential aspect of practicing autosuggestion is to refrain from engaging the will. Unlike traditional methods where willpower is utilized to achieve goals, autosuggestion operates differently. If your will conflicts with the imagination—if, for instance, you think, *"I will make such and such a thing happen,"* while your imagination responds, *"You are willing it, but it is not going to be"*—you not only fail to attain your desired outcome, but you may even experience the opposite result.

"When practicing autosuggestion, it's crucial to align your thoughts with your imagination and avoid imposing your will upon the process."

This harmonious synchronization between thought and imagination is the key to unlocking the transformative potential of autosuggestion.

The insight provided here is crucial and sheds light on why traditional approaches focusing solely on re-educating the will often yield unsatisfactory results in treating moral ailments. Instead, the key lies in training the imagination. This nuanced distinction is what has enabled the Coué method to succeed where others have failed.

Emile Coué

"Drawing from two decades of daily experimentation and meticulous examination, I've formulated the following conclusions, which I've categorized as laws:"

> *"When there's a conflict between the will and the imagination, it's invariably the imagination that prevails, without exception."*

> *"In this conflict, the power of the imagination is directly proportional to the square of the will."*

"When the will and the imagination are aligned, they don't merely add to each other; rather, they multiply each other's effectiveness.

Crucially, the imagination can be directed."

"While the expressions *"in direct ratio to the square of the will"* and *"is multiplied by"* are not strictly precise, they serve as illustrative tools to clarify my intended meaning."

Given these insights, it might seem that nobody should suffer from illness. Indeed, every ailment has the potential to succumb to autosuggestion. However, it's important to note that while autosuggestion can be effective, it's not a guarantee of success in every case.

To encourage individuals to practice conscious autosuggestion, they must be taught how to do so—much like learning to read, write, or play the piano.

Autosuggestion is an innate instrument we possess from birth, akin to a baby's instinctual play with a rattle. Yet, it's a double-edged sword: handled unconsciously and imprudently, it can cause harm or even prove fatal. Conversely, when employed consciously, it has the potential to save lives.

"In the words of Aesop regarding the tongue, it can be both the best and the worst thing in the world."

Now, I'll demonstrate how anyone can benefit from the positive effects of consciously applied autosuggestion. While I say *"everyone,"* it's important to acknowledge that there are exceptions—two distinct groups in whom arousing conscious autosuggestion is challenging:

> ***The mentally undeveloped:*** Individuals who lack the cognitive capacity to comprehend the instructions or suggestions given to them.
>
> ***Those who are unwilling to understand:*** Individuals who resist or refuse to grasp the concepts or techniques of conscious autosuggestion, perhaps due to skepticism, stubbornness, or other personal reasons.

For these two groups, achieving the desired results through conscious autosuggestion may prove difficult or even impossible. However, for the vast majority of individuals, embracing and applying conscious autosuggestion can unlock a multitude of benefits and transformative outcomes.

How to Teach Patients to Make Autosuggestions

Teaching patients to utilize autosuggestions is grounded in a fundamental principle: our minds have difficulty simultaneously holding conflicting thoughts. When a singular idea dominates our mental landscape, it shapes our reality and propels us toward corresponding actions. Thoughts breed emotions, which in turn prompt behaviors, leading to physical sensations that reinforce those initial thoughts. In Cognitive Behavioral Therapy (CBT), this interconnected loop is often referred to as the five Ps or the vicious cycle.

For instance, if you can convince a sick person that their condition is improving, their illness may indeed diminish. Similarly, if a kleptomaniac sincerely believes they will no longer steal, they are likely to cease their thieving behavior.

While this training may initially appear daunting, it's actually quite straightforward. Through a series of carefully crafted and progressively challenging exercises, patients can be guided through the basics of conscious thought. Here's the step-by-step process:

- ❖ Start with simple, manageable suggestions and gradually increase their complexity.
- ❖ Ensure that each suggestion is tailored to the individual's specific circumstances and challenges.
- ❖ Encourage patients to fully immerse themselves in each suggestion, allowing it to occupy their entire mental space.

❖ Repeat the process consistently, reinforcing positive suggestions over time.

By following this structured approach diligently, one can expect to achieve positive outcomes in most cases, barring the exceptions mentioned earlier. It's important to note that while this method may seem simplistic, its efficacy lies in its simplicity and systematic application.

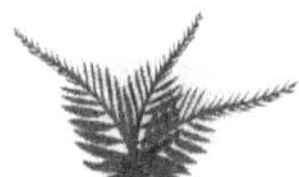

The first experiment involves a preparatory phase followed by a physical demonstration. Here's how to conduct it:

Preparatory Phase:
- Instruct the subject to stand upright, maintaining a rigid posture with the body as stiff as an iron bar.
- Ensure that the subject's feet are positioned close together, aligned from toe to heel, while keeping the ankles flexible as if they were hinges.
- Explain to the subject that they should imagine themselves as a plank balanced on the ground, with hinges at its base.
- Demonstrate how a plank falls easily when pushed slightly in any direction without resistance.
- Inform the subject that you will gently pull them backward by the shoulders, and they must allow themselves to fall into your arms without resisting, maintaining their feet fixed to the ground and pivoting on their ankles like hinges.

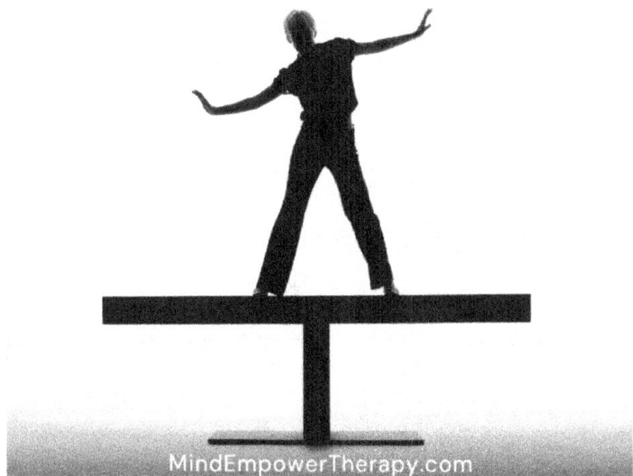

Physical Demonstration:

- Pull the subject backward by the shoulders, applying gentle force.
- Encourage the subject to relax and allow themselves to fall into your arms, maintaining their feet firmly planted on the ground and pivoting on their ankles.
- Repeat the experiment as necessary until the subject successfully executes the movement without resistance or hesitation.

This experiment is attributed to the Sage of Rochester and serves as an initial step in demonstrating the power of suggestion and bodily response. Through repetition and reinforcement, subjects can gradually learn to overcome resistance and respond more fluidly to suggestions.

The second experiment aims to illustrate the influence of imagination on bodily responses. Here's how to conduct it:

Preparation:

- Explain to the subject that you will demonstrate how their imagination can influence their physical sensations.
- Instruct the subject to focus solely on the thought: "I am falling backwards, I am falling backwards." Emphasize that they should not entertain any other thoughts, doubts, or concerns during the experiment.
- Ensure that the subject understands not to resist the impulse to fall if they genuinely feel compelled to do so.

Execution:

- Ask the subject to stand with their head held high and eyes closed.
- Position your right fist on the back of the subject's neck and your left hand on their forehead.
- Begin verbally instructing the subject: "Now, think: 'I am falling backwards, I am falling backwards,'" while simultaneously sliding your left hand lightly backward to the left temple, above the ear.
- As you continue to repeat the suggestion, slowly remove your right fist from the back of the subject's neck in a smooth, continuous motion.

During this process, maintain a calm and reassuring demeanor to help the subject feel comfortable and open to the suggestion. It's essential to monitor the subject's response closely and ensure their safety throughout the experiment.

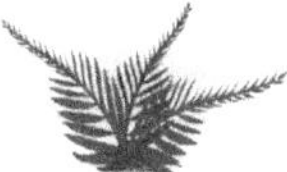

After the subject makes a slight movement backward, one of two outcomes may occur: they may either stop themselves from falling or they may fall completely. If the subject resists falling, explain to them that their resistance was likely due to thoughts of potential harm if they were to fall. Emphasize that had they not entertained such thoughts, they would have fallen effortlessly.

To address this resistance, repeat the experiment with a commanding tone, as if you are compelling the subject to obey your instructions without hesitation. Continue conducting the experiment until it is successfully executed, or until the subject is very close to falling.

It's crucial for the operator to stand slightly behind the subject, with the left leg forward and the right leg well behind, to avoid being knocked over in case the subject falls backward. Neglecting this precaution could result in both the subject and the operator falling, especially if the subject is heavy. Safety should always be prioritized during the experiment.

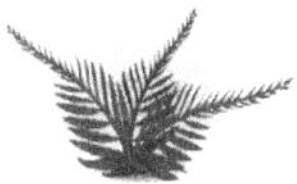

The third experiment focuses on inducing the sensation of falling forward. Here's how to conduct it:

Positioning:

- Have the subject face you with their body stiff, ankles flexible, and feet joined and parallel.
- Place your hands lightly on the subject's temples without applying any pressure.

Instruction:

- Instruct the subject to maintain their gaze fixed on a point at the root of their nose without moving their eyelids.
- Prompt the subject to think: "I am falling forward, I am falling forward," while emphasizing each syllable. Repeat the suggestion verbally, saying, "You are fall . . . ing . . . for . . . ward, You are fall . . . ing . . . for . . . ward," while maintaining steady eye contact without blinking.

During the experiment, ensure that the subject remains relaxed and receptive to the suggestion. Continue to repeat the instructions and maintain eye contact until the desired sensation is induced or until the subject experiences a noticeable response. As with previous experiments, prioritize the subject's safety and well-being throughout the process.

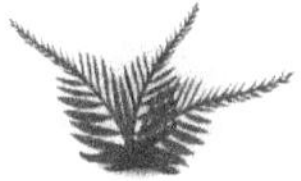

The fourth experiment demonstrates the power of suggestion in influencing physical actions. Here are the steps to conduct it:

Preparation:

- Instruct the subject to clasp their hands together as tightly as possible until their fingers tremble slightly.
- Maintain eye contact with the subject in the same manner as in the previous experiment, while keeping your hands on theirs as if to squeeze them together even more tightly.

Instruction:

- Prompt the subject to think that they cannot unclasp their fingers, emphasizing the idea that they are unable to do so.
- Inform the subject that you will count to three, and when you say *"three,"* they should attempt to separate their hands while continuously thinking, *"I cannot do it, I cannot do it."*
- Count slowly, *"one, two, three,"* and immediately add, detached syllables, *"You . . . can . . . not . . . do . . . it. . . . You . . . can . . . not . . . do . . . it. . . ."*

During this process, if the subject is properly focused on the thought *"I cannot do it,"* they will find it impossible to separate their fingers. In fact, their fingers may clasp together even more tightly with each effort to separate them, achieving the opposite of what they intend. This demonstrates the influence of autosuggestion on physical actions.

To conclude the experiment, instruct the subject to think, *"I can do it,"* and they will find that their fingers will separate themselves. This experiment highlights the profound effect of suggestion on the body's responses and reinforces the principles of conscious autosuggestion.

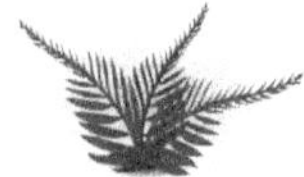

During the fourth experiment, it's crucial to maintain strict control over the subject and ensure their compliance with the instructions. Here are some additional guidelines:

Eye Contact:

- Keep your gaze fixed on the root of the subject's nose throughout the experiment.
- Prevent the subject from diverting their eyes away from yours at any point.

Reinforcement:

- If the subject is unable to unclasp their hands, reinforce the idea that it is their own failure to properly focus on the thought "I cannot."
- Assure the subject firmly that any lack of success is solely their responsibility, not yours.

Tone of Command:

- Maintain a tone of command throughout the experiment, conveying authority and expecting complete obedience.
- Use a firm and authoritative tone without necessarily raising your voice. Emphasize each word distinctly to convey the seriousness of the instructions.

By adhering to these guidelines, you can ensure that the subject remains focused and compliant, maximizing the effectiveness of the experiment and reinforcing the principles of autosuggestion.

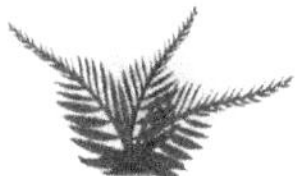

Once the initial experiments have proven successful, further exercises can be performed with ease, following the same principles outlined earlier. Here are some additional considerations:

Sensitivity of Subjects:
- Some subjects may exhibit heightened sensitivity, easily responding to suggestions with physical reactions such as finger or limb contractions.
- Recognize these sensitive individuals, as their responses indicate a strong susceptibility to autosuggestion.

Simplified Instructions:
- After a few successful experiments, there's no need to explicitly instruct the subjects to "think this" or "think that."
- Instead, give straightforward commands using the imperative tone commonly used in suggestion techniques. For example:
  - "Close your hands; now you cannot open them."
  - "Shut your eyes; now you cannot open them."

Results:

- Subjects will find it absolutely impossible to open their hands or eyes, despite their efforts, when given such commands.
- After a brief period, inform the subject that they can now perform the action, and they will de-contract instantaneously, regaining control over their hands or eyes.

By adapting the instructions to the sensitivity and responsiveness of the subjects, you can effectively demonstrate the power of autosuggestion and further reinforce its principles.

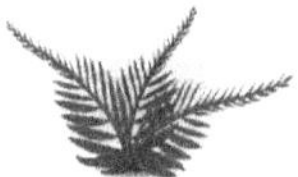

These experiments can be endlessly varied to explore the depths of autosuggestion. Here are a few more examples:

Welded Hands:
- Instruct the subject to join their hands, suggesting that they are welded together seamlessly.

Stuck Hand:
- Have the subject place their hand on a table, then suggest that it is firmly stuck to the surface.

Fixed to Chair:
- Tell the subject that they are firmly fixed to their chair and incapable of rising from it.

Immobility:

- Instruct the subject to rise from their chair, then suggest that they are unable to move or walk.

Heavy Object:
- Place a penholder on the table and suggest to the subject that it weighs an enormous amount, making it impossible for them to lift.

These experiments are not simply about suggestion alone. It's essential to emphasize that the phenomena observed are not solely a result of the operator's suggestion but rather the subsequent autosuggestion generated within the subject's mind.

By delving into these variations, we continue to uncover the profound influence of autosuggestion on our thoughts, behaviors, and physical responses. Each experiment serves to illuminate the power of the mind to shape our reality through the process of autosuggestion.

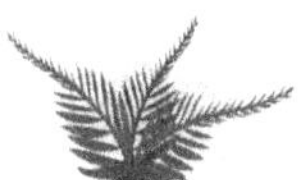

To illustrate the power of autosuggestion, Coué frequently relies on a set of examples that highlight the weakness of conscious will in comparison to the imagination:

The Insomnia Example: Coué points out that when individuals try too hard to fall asleep, they often end up staying awake. Additionally, he could have mentioned that believing in the effectiveness of a placebo sleeping tablet can actually lead to falling asleep.

The Forgetting Example: People often struggle to remember something, but the more they try, the more elusive the memory becomes. Yet, when they stop trying, the information often spontaneously comes back to them.

The Laughter Example: Coué notes that attempts to suppress laughter often result in intensified giggling. This phenomenon mirrors the experience of actors "corpsing" on stage, unable to control their laughter.

The Cycling Example: When individuals learn to ride a bike and focus too much on avoiding obstacles, they often lose balance and crash. Similarly, people struggling to swim may sink instead of calmly staying afloat.

The Stammering Example: Individuals who stutter may find that their speech worsens when they become anxious about it. Yet, when they practice alone, their speech may be fluent.

The "Walking the Plank" Example: Coué uses Pascal's analogy of walking across a plank on the ground versus one suspended high above. The fear of falling interferes with the ability to perform a simple task, illustrating the conflict between will and imagination.

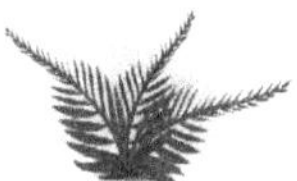

Summing up these examples, Coué concludes emphatically:

"Every time the WILL and the IMAGINATION clash, not only do we fail to achieve our desired outcome, but we often achieve the opposite."

These examples serve as compelling rhetorical tools, resonating with various audiences due to their simplicity and universality.

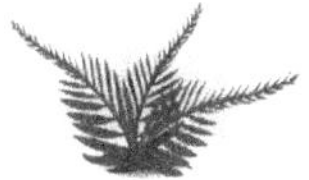

The "Cue-Controlled Tension-Release CD Script"

The "Cue-Controlled Tension-Release CD Script" is designed to guide individuals through a process of becoming more aware of tension in their bodies and learning to release it through controlled muscle relaxation. Let's see a breakdown of the script:

Preamble:

- Encourages the individual to get comfortable and relax deeply before beginning.
- Explains the purpose of the exercise: to become more aware of tension in the body and learn to relax more deeply.

Rationale:

- Explains the importance of becoming aware of muscle tension and learning to relax.
- Assures the individual that it's normal to fall asleep during the exercise and emphasizes the importance of relaxation.

Motivation:

- Highlights the potential benefits of learning to relax muscles, such as reducing stress and improving health.
- Encourages the individual to focus on their body and prepare for the main exercise.

Muscle Tension and Release:

- Guides the individual through tense and release exercises for various muscle groups, starting with the arms, shoulders, forehead, face, jaw, and legs.
- Emphasizes studying the sensations of tension and relaxation during each exercise.
- Encourages the individual to relax completely after each tension phase and notice the contrast between tension and relaxation.

Imagination:

- Guides the individual through an exercise where they imagine tension in their body without physically tensing the muscles.
- Encourages the individual to notice any tension that arises during the imagination exercise and release it.

Counting:

- Guides the individual through a deep relaxation exercise, counting down from five to zero while encouraging deeper relaxation with each count.

Deep Breaths & Verbal Cue:

- Guides the individual through deep breathing exercises while repeating the word "RELAX" in their mind.
- Encourages the individual to use a verbal cue (e.g., saying "RELAX" mentally) to signal relaxation.

Conclusion:

- Encourages the individual to note their peak relaxation level and remain aware of muscle tension throughout the day.
- Guides the individual through a gradual return to wakefulness, counting up from one to five and encouraging movement and deep breathing.
- Congratulates the individual on completing the exercise and encourages them to remain calm and relaxed in their daily activities.

Overall, the script aims to help individuals develop awareness of muscle tension and learn effective relaxation techniques for stress management.

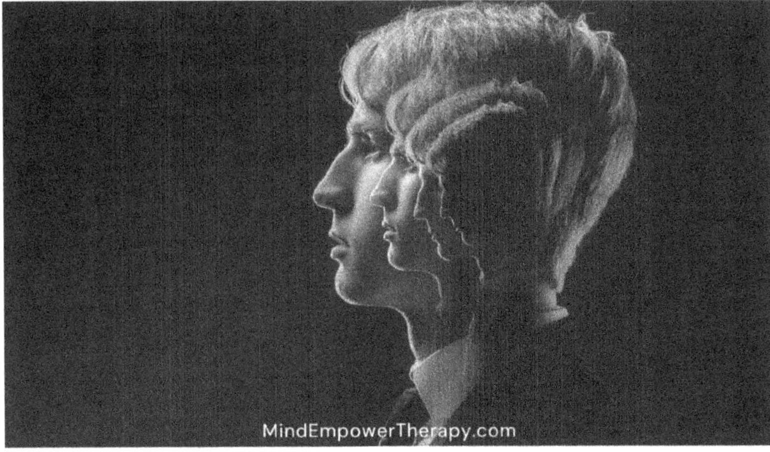

Unforgettable Practical Experiments by Coué!

---

1. The Hand Clasp Experiment:

Subjects are instructed to tightly clasp their hands together and extend their arms. They are then directed to repeat to themselves, often rapidly and under their breath, "I will open my hands, but I CANNOT, I CANNOT!" Coué intensifies the suggestion by emphasizing, "Your hands lock tighter and tighter, always tighter!" This suggestion is reinforced, implying that the hands cannot be separated by effort as long as the contrary idea persists in the imagination. After a brief pause, the subjects are instructed to change their self-talk to "I CAN!" while imagining they can indeed separate their hands. This test has become a staple in hypnotic demonstrations, resembling the concept of self-efficacy statements in Bandura's research.

2. The Postural Sway Experiment:

Subjects stand rigidly and tense, like a plank, and suggest to themselves that they are falling forward or backward, to be caught by a practitioner.

3. The Fist-Clench Experiment:

Subjects clench their fists and suggest to themselves that their fists cannot open. After an initial effort, they shift their self-talk to believe that their fists can open again.

4. The Pen-Drop Experiment:

Subjects grasp a pen between their fingers and suggest to themselves that they cannot release it. Practitioner asks them to imagine that the more they try to drop it, the tighter their fingers grasp, until they imagine their fingers releasing.

5. The Hand Stuck Experiment:

Subjects press their palm onto a tabletop and suggest that it is stuck in place and cannot be lifted.

6. The Stiff Leg Experiment:

Subjects imagine their legs are stiff and stuck in place, rendering them unable to walk.

7. The Stuck in Chair Experiment:

Subjects imagine being glued to their chair, preventing them from standing up.

Coué also references the well-known **"sucking a lemon"** experiment, where subjects visualize sucking a lemon and notice their mouth salivating. This simple example illustrates the **ideo-reflex response or the effect of autosuggestion and imagination** on the body's autonomic processes.

These techniques involve either autosuggestions of a single muscular movement or two antagonistic muscular responses, inducing a cataleptic response to challenges resisting the original dominant idea. Baudouin favored Chevreul's famous **"exploratory pendulum"** experiment, finding it effective due to its inherent amplification of the **ideo-motor response** and simple movement.

Highlights from Coué's Seminar Conclusion

It is important to understand that Coué reinforced the importance of understanding autosuggestion for its effective application. He believed that the success of these techniques rested on the individual's readiness and willingness to engage with them, emphasizing the need for preparation and confidence in one's ability to influence the mind and body.

Coué always concluded his seminars by instructing his subjects to close their eyes, acknowledging that despite rejecting the label of *"self-hypnosis,"* closing the eyes and relaxing helps focus the mind on the imagination. He then delivers a series of positive suggestions for the entire group, to be repeated internally by each individual. Beginning with a graceful reassurance that his suggestions, with their consent, will be permanently fixed in their minds and positively affect **"the whole organism,"** Coué sets the tone for a traditional hypnosis script focused on general physical well-being and healthy functioning.

The climax of his session features a powerful statement of self-efficacy or **"ego-strengthening,"** where he declares:

"Finally and above all, and this is most essential for everyone, if up to the present you have felt a certain distrust of yourself, this distrust from now onwards will gradually disappear, and will give place to a feeling of confidence in yourself. **YOU WILL HAVE CONFIDENCE IN YOURSELF, you hear me, YOU WILL HAVE CONFIDENCE IN YOURSELF**. I repeat it, and this confidence will enable you to do whatever you want to do well, even very well, whatever it may be, on condition, naturally, that it is reasonable […]."

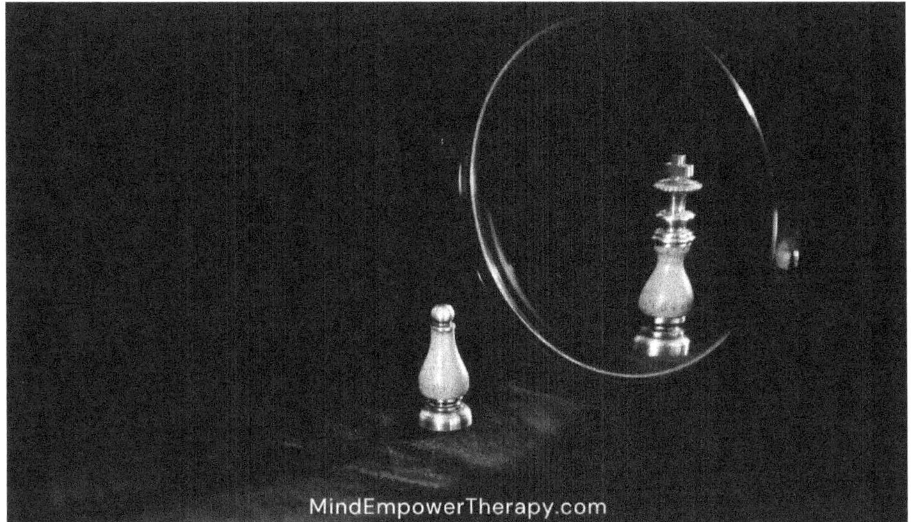

He also emphasizes the belief that what one wishes to do is easy, making it so for them, even if it appears difficult to others. This confidence, he asserts, facilitates quick and proficient task completion, devoid of fatigue or effort. Conversely, deeming a task difficult or impossible would only make it so, simply because one thought it to be.

While modern hypnotists prioritize focusing on solutions, briefly mentioning problems or mistakes before transitioning to a more positive outcome, the impact of Coué's seminars undoubtedly left participants with an impressive sense of the potential of autosuggestion.

Mastering the Script Method of Curative Suggestion

Once the subject has successfully navigated the preliminary experiments and comprehended their implications, they are ready for the transformative potential of curative suggestion. At this stage, they resemble a fertile field where seeds can take root and flourish, whereas previously, they were akin to untamed terrain where seeds would have withered away.

Regardless of the ailment afflicting the subject, be it physical or mental, it is crucial to adhere to a consistent method and employ similar language, albeit with minor adjustments tailored to the specific case at hand. This uniform approach ensures clarity and effectiveness in delivering curative suggestions.

Say to the subject: "Sit down and close your eyes. I am not going to try to put you to sleep as it is unnecessary. Close your eyes simply so that your attention may not be distracted by the objects around you. Now, tell yourself that every word I say is going to firmly embed itself in your mind, becoming deeply ingrained and integrated within it. It will be fixed, imprinted, and encrusted there, without your conscious will or knowledge. Your entire being, including your organism, will obey these suggestions effortlessly and unconsciously.

Firstly, I instruct you that every day, three times a day—morning, noon, and evening, coinciding with your usual meal times—you will feel hungry.

You will experience the pleasant sensation that prompts you to think and say, 'Oh! How delightful it will be to have something to eat!' You will then consume your food with enjoyment, being careful not to overeat. Ensure that you chew your food thoroughly, transforming it into a soft paste before swallowing. Under these conditions, you will digest your food properly, experiencing no discomfort, inconvenience, or pain whatsoever in your stomach or intestines. You will efficiently assimilate the nutrients, and your organism will utilize them to produce blood, muscle, strength, and energy—essentially, sustaining your life."

Since you will have digested your food properly, your excretory function will be normal. Each morning upon rising, you will feel the natural urge to evacuate your bowels. Without any need for medication or artificial aids, you will achieve a normal and satisfactory result.

Furthermore, every night, from the moment you decide to go to sleep until the time you wish to wake the next morning, you will experience deep, peaceful sleep without any disturbances or nightmares. Upon awakening, you will feel perfectly refreshed, cheerful, and full of energy to start your day.

Similarly, if you occasionally experience feelings of depression, gloominess, and tend to focus on the negative aspects of life, from now on, you will cease to do so. Instead of feeling worried and depressed, you will feel perfectly cheerful, perhaps without any specific reason, just as you previously felt down without a particular cause. Furthermore, even if there are genuine reasons for concern and depression, you will not succumb to such feelings.

Moreover, if you sometimes find yourself succumbing to impatience or irritability, those tendencies will disappear. Instead, you will remain patient and in control of yourself at all times. The things that used to bother, irritate, or upset you will no longer have any effect on you, and you will remain completely calm and indifferent to them.

Additionally, if you are occasionally troubled by negative and unhealthy thoughts, fears, aversions, temptations, or resentments towards others, all of those will gradually fade away from your imagination. They will dissipate and vanish like a distant cloud, eventually disappearing completely. Just as a dream fades away upon waking, these vain images will fade from your mind.

All your bodily organs are functioning properly. Your heart beats in a normal rhythm, and your blood circulation occurs as it should. Your lungs are carrying out their functions effectively, as are your stomach, intestines, liver, biliary duct, kidneys, and bladder. If any of these organs are currently experiencing abnormalities, those irregularities are diminishing every day, and soon they will disappear entirely, restoring the organ to its normal function. Moreover, if there are any lesions present in any of these organs, they will progressively improve each day until they are completely healed.

It's important to note that it's not necessary to identify which specific organ is affected for it to be healed. Through the influence of the autosuggestion **"Every day, in every way, I am getting better and better,"** your unconscious mind acts upon the organ in need of healing, identifying and addressing the issue without conscious intervention.

It is crucial to emphasize that if you have lacked confidence in yourself until now, I assure you that this self-doubt will gradually fade away, replaced by a sense of self-assurance rooted in the understanding of the immense power within each of us. It is absolutely essential for every individual to possess this self-confidence, as without it, one can achieve nothing, whereas with it, one can accomplish whatever they desire (within reasonable limits, of course).

You will develop confidence in yourself, and this newfound confidence will provide you with the certainty that you are fully capable of achieving whatever you set out to do—provided it is reasonable and aligns with your responsibilities.

Therefore, whenever you embark on a reasonable task or have a duty to fulfill, always approach it with the mindset that it is easy. Banish from your vocabulary words like "difficult," "impossible," "I cannot," or "it is stronger than I." These words are not reflective of the English language. Instead, focus on affirmations such as "It is easy, and I can do it." By perceiving the task as easy, it will indeed become easy for you, even if it may appear challenging to others. You will accomplish it swiftly and proficiently, without experiencing fatigue, because you approach it effortlessly. Conversely, if you were to view the task as difficult or impossible, it would become so for you simply because you believed it to be so.

In addition to these comprehensive suggestions, which may appear lengthy or simplistic to some, but are indeed essential, specific suggestions tailored to the individual patient must also be included.

These suggestions should be delivered in a monotone and calming voice, with emphasis on key words. While this delivery does not induce actual sleep, it does induce a drowsy state in the subject, causing them to think of nothing in particular.

When you have completed the series of suggestions, you address the subject as follows: **"In summary, I mean that from every aspect, both physical and mental, you will enjoy excellent health, better than what you have experienced so far. Now, I am going to count to three, and when I say 'Three, you will open your eyes and emerge from the passive state you are in. You will come out of it naturally, without feeling drowsy or tired. On the contrary, you will feel strong, alert, active, and full of life. Moreover, you will feel cheerful and fit in every way. 'ONE--TWO--THREE-"** At the word 'three,' the subject opens their eyes, always with a smile and an expression of well-being and contentment on their face.

Occasionally, although rarely, the patient is cured immediately. More commonly, however, the patient experiences relief; their pain or depression may partially or completely disappear, albeit temporarily.

In every case, it is necessary to administer the suggestions at varying intervals according to the needs of the subject. These suggestions should be spaced out progressively longer as the patient progresses, until they are no longer required, indicating that the cure is complete.

Before dismissing your patient, you must explain to them that they possess the instrument with which they can heal themselves, and that you are merely a teacher instructing them on how to use this instrument. You should emphasize that they must collaborate with you in this process.

Therefore, every morning upon waking and every night before going to sleep, they should close their eyes and mentally place themselves in your presence. Then, using a string with twenty knots as a counting aid, they should repeat twenty times consecutively in a monotonous voice the following phrase: **"EVERY DAY, IN EVERY WAY, I AM GETTING BETTER AND BETTER."** They should emphasize the words **"in every way,"** as this applies to all their needs, whether mental or physical. This general suggestion is more effective than specific ones.

This illustrates the role of the provider of suggestions. They are not an authoritarian figure giving commands, but rather a friend, a guide, leading the patient step by step on the path to health. Since all suggestions are given for the benefit of the patient, their unconscious mind is eager to assimilate them and transform them into autosuggestions. Once this is accomplished, the cure is achieved, the speed of which varies depending on the circumstances.

The Superiority of This Method

This method consistently produces remarkable results, and its effectiveness is easily understandable. By following the prescribed steps, failure is virtually impossible. Conversely, attempting to induce subjects into a state of hypnosis immediately, without the necessary explanations and preparatory experiments to make them receptive to suggestions and to convert them into autosuggestions, will likely lead to failure, except in the case of particularly sensitive individuals, who are rare. However, with the proper training, anyone can become sensitive to suggestions. Yet, without the preliminary instructions and exercises advocated in this method, which can be completed in a matter of minutes, success is unlikely.

By assuring the patient that sleep is unnecessary and that there is no need to induce it, trust and confidence are fostered. The patient listens attentively without fear or apprehension, and it often happens—perhaps not immediately, but eventually—that, lulled by the soothing monotony of my voice, in occasions, they drift into a deep sleep from which they awaken surprised at having slept at all.

Indeed, it's essential not to assume that autosuggestion can only occur through the specific methods I've outlined. Suggestions can be made to individuals without their awareness or any prior preparation. For example, a doctor, merely by virtue of their title, wields a suggestive influence over their patient. If that doctor tells the patient that nothing can be done for their condition, suggesting it's incurable, they may inadvertently provoke an autosuggestion in the patient's mind, leading to potentially disastrous consequences. However, if the doctor informs the patient that while their illness is serious, with careful management, time, and patience, it can be cured, they may often achieve surprising results.

Here's another example: If a doctor, after examining a patient, writes a prescription and hands it to them without any explanation, the prescribed remedies are unlikely to succeed. However, if the doctor takes the time to explain to the patient how and when to take the medications, along with the expected results, those outcomes are much more likely to be achieved.

If there are medical professionals or pharmacists in this audience, I hope they won't see me as their adversary. On the contrary, I consider myself their ally. I advocate for the inclusion of both the theoretical and practical study of suggestion in medical school curricula, for the benefit of both patients and doctors alike. Additionally, I believe that every time a patient visits their doctor, the doctor should prescribe one or even several medications, even if they aren't strictly necessary. After all, when a patient seeks medical advice, they expect to receive a prescription for medicine. They often overlook the importance of lifestyle changes and dietary adjustments, placing greater emphasis on pharmaceutical solutions.

In my view, if a doctor only prescribes lifestyle changes or dietary adjustments without any medication, the patient may feel dissatisfied. They might believe that they didn't receive proper treatment and could even seek advice from another doctor. Therefore, I believe it's important for doctors to prescribe medications to their patients whenever possible. Moreover, it's preferable for doctors to prescribe medications that they have prepared themselves rather than relying solely on commercially available remedies that are heavily advertised. Patients are likely to have greater confidence in medications prescribed directly by their doctor compared to generic pills available over the counter at any pharmacy.

How Suggestion Works

To better understand how suggestions work, let's have a close view of Coué's philosophy. Coué implicitly recognized the significance of **ideo-motor action**, which Baudouin terms as **"ideo-reflex,"** referring to the physiological process through which the imagination influences certain physical processes. He succinctly captured this concept by stating, **"Every thought entirely filling our mind becomes true for us and tends to transform itself into action" (Coué, 1922: 15)**. To illustrate the conflict between willpower and imagination, Coué conducted a series of standardized **"waking suggestion"** experiments, a practice now commonly employed in modern stage hypnosis and clinical hypnotherapy.

Describing his approach in vibrant terms, Coué likened his explanations and demonstrations to tilling the soil of his audience's minds, preparing them for the seeds of therapeutic autosuggestion (Coué, 1923: 124). He understood the vital role of his performance in instilling confidence in his audience's ability to influence their minds and bodies. For individuals to derive benefits from the method, they must grasp the concept of autosuggestion, and Coué's demonstrations played a pivotal role in this regard.

It is evident that those who have merely read about the Coué method may struggle to make it effective, as they may not have adequately prepared themselves. Coué recognized that individuals who respond positively to suggestion tests are likely to have understood how to employ autosuggestion effectively and are ready to implement it in their lives.

Understanding the workings of suggestion, or more precisely autosuggestion, is quite simple when we recognize that our unconscious mind is the ultimate director of all our bodily functions. When we convey to the unconscious that a particular organ needs to function properly, it immediately transmits the command. The organ obediently follows suit, gradually or immediately performing its functions in a normal manner. This straightforward explanation elucidates how suggestion can effectively halt hemorrhages, alleviate constipation, eliminate fibrous tumors, treat paralysis, heal tubercular lesions, address varicose veins, ulcers, and numerous other conditions.

In one occasion, Coué illustrated the power of suggestion in controlling bodily functions. In that case, a young lady was scheduled to have a tooth extracted, and Coué offered to assist her in feeling no pain during the procedure. With her consent, Coué proceeded to the dentist's office. While standing opposite her, he directed focused suggestions, repeating phrases like **"You feel nothing, you feel nothing,"** and signaled to the dentist to begin the extraction. Remarkably, the tooth was removed swiftly without any apparent discomfort to the patient. However, as sometimes occurs, a hemorrhage ensued after the extraction.

Opting to utilize suggestion rather than a hemostatic agent, Coué instructed the dentist not to intervene and proceeded to suggest to the patient that the hemorrhage would cease spontaneously in two minutes. With the patient's attention fixed on Coué, they waited, and after a brief period, the bleeding stopped on its own. Upon examination, they observed a clot of blood had formed in the dental cavity, effectively resolving the hemorrhage without any external intervention.

The phenomenon can be explained simply: under the influence of the suggestion that the hemorrhage is to stop, the unconscious mind sends instructions to the small arteries and veins to halt the flow of blood. In response, these blood vessels contract naturally, just as they would in reaction to a hemostatic agent like adrenaline.

Similarly, the disappearance of a fibrous tumor can be understood in the same way. When the unconscious accepts the idea that the tumor is to go, the brain commands the arteries supplying it to contract. As a result, these arteries cease to nourish the tumor, causing it to lose its source of sustenance. Consequently, the tumor dies, dries up, is reabsorbed, and eventually disappears.

The Definitive Guide to Essential Cures

Coué emphasizes...

This little work would be incomplete if it did not include a few examples of the cures obtained. It would take too long, and would also perhaps be somewhat tiring if I were to relate all those in which I have taken part. I will therefore content myself by quoting a few of the most remarkable.

Mlle. M---- D----, a resident of Troyes, endured the torment of asthma for a staggering eight years. Nights were a battleground for her, as she struggled to catch her breath while propped up in bed. Recognizing her sensitivity, we initiated preliminary experiments, during which she readily fell into a deep slumber. With the application of suggestion during these sessions, we witnessed remarkable progress. Following the first treatment, there was a remarkable improvement. She enjoyed a restful night, with only a brief quarter-hour episode of asthma interrupting her sleep. In a remarkably short span, her asthma vanished entirely, with no recurrence in the future.

M. M----, a working hosier residing in Sainte-Savine near Troyes, endured paralysis for a staggering two years due to injuries at the junction of the spinal column and the pelvis. The paralysis was confined to his lower limbs, which exhibited severely impaired blood circulation, resulting in swelling, congestion, and discoloration. Despite several attempted treatments, including antisyphilitic measures, none proved successful. Preliminary experiments demonstrated success, prompting the application of suggestion by me and autosuggestion by the patient for eight days. At the conclusion of this period, there was a slight but discernible movement in the left leg. With renewed suggestion, there was noticeable improvement within eight days. Subsequently, progress continued, with gradual reduction of swelling and other symptoms. Eleven months later, on November 1, 1906, the patient accomplished the remarkable feat of descending stairs unassisted and walking a distance of 800 yards. By July 1907, he had returned to his factory job, displaying no lingering traces of paralysis.

M. A---- G----, residing in Troyes, had long grappled with enteritis, despite numerous unsuccessful treatments. Additionally, he battled severe mental distress, characterized by depression, desolation, social withdrawal, and suicidal thoughts. Preliminary experiments indicated favorable conditions, prompting the application of suggestion which yielded tangible results from the outset. Over the course of three months, daily suggestions were administered initially, followed by gradually spaced intervals. By the end of this period, the cure was comprehensive: the enteritis had vanished, and his demeanor had undergone a remarkable transformation. Twelve years later, with no signs of relapse, the cure is deemed permanent. M. G---- serves as a compelling illustration of the efficacy of suggestion, or more accurately, autosuggestion. Concurrently addressing both physical and mental aspects, he embraced the suggestions with equal efficacy. His self-confidence surged daily, leading him to seek opportunities for professional advancement. Recognizing his exceptional skills, an employer provided him with the desired machinery to work from home. Capitalizing on his proficiency, M. G---- exceeded ordinary productivity levels, prompting his employer to entrust him with additional machinery. Thus, what would have been an ordinary workman, owing to suggestion, evolved into a supervisor managing six machines, yielding substantial profits.

Mme. D----, residing in Troyes and approximately 30 years old, was in the advanced stages of consumption, with her condition deteriorating daily despite specialized nourishment. Afflicted with persistent coughing, spitting, and breathing difficulties, her prognosis seemed bleak, suggesting she had only a few months left to live. Preliminary experiments indicated considerable sensitivity, and suggestion elicited immediate improvement. Remarkably, from the following day, her morbid symptoms began to subside. With each passing day, her recovery became more pronounced, and she swiftly regained weight, even without the need for specialized nourishment. Within a few months, the cure appeared to be complete. In a letter dated January 1, 1911, eight months after my departure from Troyes, she expressed her gratitude and reported that, despite being pregnant, she was in perfect health.

Before I conclude, I'd like to touch on the application of my method to the upbringing and guidance of children by their parents.

Parents should wait until their child is asleep, then one of them should enter the child's room quietly, stopping a short distance from the bed. They should softly repeat 15 or 20 times the things they wish to instill in the child, concerning health, diligence, sleep, behavior, and so on. Afterward, they should leave the room just as quietly, taking care not to wake the child. This simple process yields remarkable results for several reasons. When a child is asleep, their body and conscious mind are at rest, but their unconscious mind remains active. Speaking directly to the unconscious mind during sleep allows suggestions to be accepted without resistance. Over time, the child naturally aligns their behavior with the desires and expectations of their parents, shaping themselves accordingly.

The key takeaway is straightforward

Within each of us lies an immense power that, when left unguided, can often work against our best interests. However, if we learn to harness and direct this power consciously and wisely, it grants us control over ourselves. With it, we can not only overcome physical and mental challenges but also lead relatively happy lives, regardless of our circumstances.

Most importantly, this power should be utilized for the moral redemption of those who have strayed from the right path.

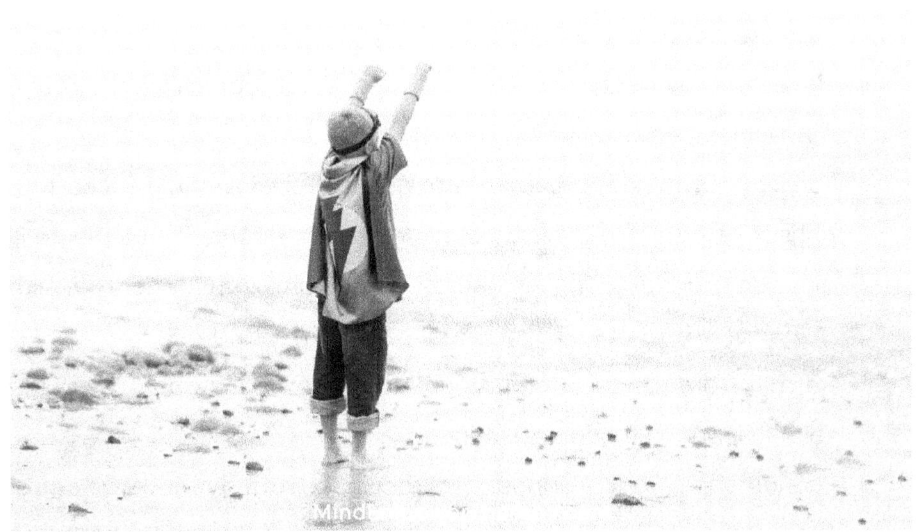

Unlocking the Power of Positive Thinking: Emile Coué's Wisdom and Inspiration

Here are invaluable thoughts and precepts of Emile Coué, as recorded by his disciple, Mme. Emile Leon you might find impiring:

"Do not waste your time dwelling on illnesses you might have, for if you do not have real ones, you will end up creating artificial ones."

- Avoid dwelling on potential illnesses, as excessive focus on them can manifest them artificially.
- When practicing conscious autosuggestion, keep it simple, natural, and firm, avoiding any strain or effort. Negative suggestions often manifest because they are made effortlessly.
- Have confidence that reasonable desires can be achieved through autosuggestion.
- To gain self-mastery, believe that you are attaining it. If faced with physical tremors or weaknesses, affirm to yourself that they will diminish gradually. Trust in your own inner strength for healing, with guidance provided to harness that power effectively.
- Refrain from discussing topics you lack knowledge about, as doing so only leads to embarrassment.
- Phenomena that appear miraculous often have natural explanations; their extraordinary nature arises from our inability to comprehend their cause. Recognizing this brings a sense of naturalness to seemingly extraordinary events.

- In conflicts between willpower and imagination, the imagination typically prevails. Attempting to force actions or suppress emotions often results in the opposite outcome. Therefore, rather than focusing on strengthening the will, it is more beneficial to train and harness the power of the imagination.

- Our perception of things is not based on their inherent nature but on how they appear to us. This discrepancy in perception can lead to contradictory accounts from individuals speaking sincerely.

- By adopting the belief that one has control over their thoughts, they indeed gain mastery over them.

- Every thought, whether positive or negative, has the power to manifest into reality. We shape our own destinies through our thoughts and actions, independent of external circumstances.

- Those who approach life with the conviction that they will succeed inevitably find success, as they actively pursue opportunities and create favorable conditions. Conversely, those who doubt themselves fail to recognize opportunities even when surrounded by them. Instead of blaming fate, individuals should take responsibility for their actions and beliefs.

- The notion of effort should be rejected, as it often leads to the interference of the imagination and results in the opposite of what is desired.

- Always approach tasks with the mindset that they are easy, as this conserves energy and prevents unnecessary expenditure of strength. Conversely, considering tasks difficult leads to wastage of energy.

- Autosuggestion is a tool that requires skillful use, akin to mastering any other instrument. Inexperienced hands may yield poor results, but with practice and skill development, one can achieve greater success.

- Conscious autosuggestion, when practiced with confidence, faith, and perseverance, manifests itself predictably, within reasonable bounds.

- Some individuals may not achieve desired results with autosuggestion due to a lack of confidence or because they exert effort, which is a common issue. Effective suggestion requires effortless execution, completely devoid of willful exertion, relying solely on the imagination.

- Many individuals who have diligently cared for their health throughout their lives may mistakenly believe that they can be instantly cured through autosuggestion. However, it is unreasonable to expect such immediate results. Autosuggestion can only deliver what is normally achievable: a gradual improvement that eventually leads to complete recovery, if possible.

- Various healing methods employed by practitioners ultimately rely on autosuggestion. Whether through words, rituals, gestures, or theatrical performances, these methods induce in the patient the suggestion of healing.

- Every physical illness is accompanied by a mental aspect, unless it is solely psychological. The mental component can vary greatly in intensity, potentially overshadowing the physical ailment. In some cases, the mental aspect can disappear instantaneously, leaving only the physical illness behind. This phenomenon, often deemed miraculous, is simply the result of autosuggestion at work.

- Contrary to common belief, physical diseases are often more easily treatable than mental ones.

- Buffon famously remarked, "Style is the man." We might add to that: "Man is what he thinks." The fear of failure tends to lead to failure, while the belief in success can bring about success, empowering individuals to overcome obstacles they encounter.
- Conviction is crucial for both the suggester and the subject. It is this unwavering belief, this faith, that enables the suggester to achieve results even when other methods have failed.
- It is not the individual who acts, but the method itself.
- Contrary to popular belief, suggestion, or autosuggestion, has the potential to heal organic lesions.
- Previously, it was thought that hypnotism could only be effective in treating nervous disorders; however, its scope extends far beyond that. While hypnotism operates through the nervous system, this system governs the entire body. Nerves control muscle movement, regulate circulation by influencing the heart and blood vessels, and impact the functioning of all organs. Therefore, through this mechanism, all unhealthy organs can be influenced. - Dr. Paul Joire, President of the Société Universelle d'Études Psychiques (Bulletin No. 4 of the S.L.P.)
- "Moral influence holds significant value as a healing aid. Neglecting it would be a grave oversight, as spiritual forces guide the world in medicine and every other human endeavor." - Dr. Louis Renon, Lecturer at the Faculty of Medicine of Paris and physician at Necker Hospital.
- "Never forget the cardinal principle of autosuggestion: maintain optimism relentlessly, even when circumstances seem to contradict it." - René de Drabois (Bulletin 11 of the S.L.P.A.)

- "Suggestion, fueled by faith, is a formidable force." - Dr. A. L., Paris (July, 1920)
- "To possess and inspire unshakable confidence, one must walk with the assurance of genuine sincerity, desiring the good of others more than one's own." - "Culture de la Force Morale" by C. Baudouin

EMILE COUÉ: Education Done Right

COUÉ believed that education should begin even before a child is born. It may seem paradoxical, but a mother's mental state during pregnancy can significantly influence the qualities of the child. If a woman, shortly after conception, forms a clear mental image of the desired sex and attributes of her child and continues to reinforce this image throughout gestation, the child is more likely to embody those qualities.

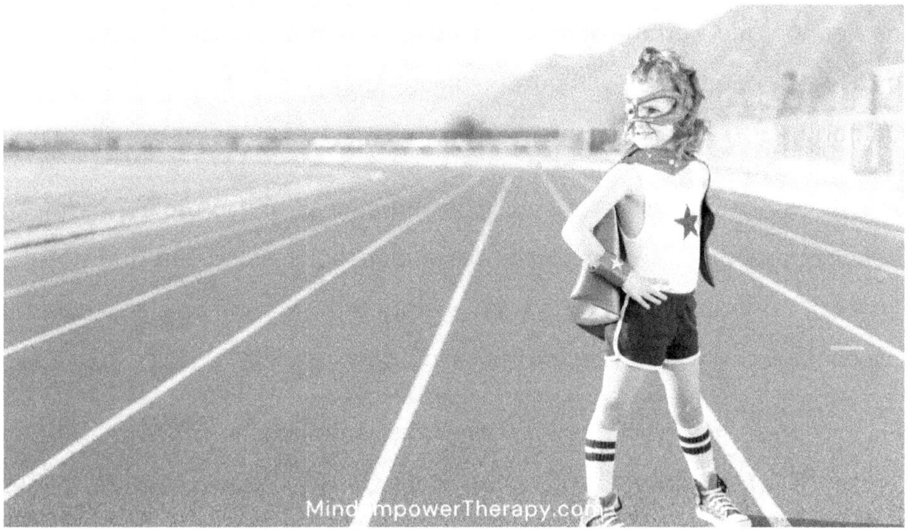

Historical examples illustrate this principle. Spartan women, desiring to contribute fierce warriors to their country, gave birth to robust children who grew up to be formidable soldiers. In contrast, Athenian mothers aimed to nurture intellectual prowess in their offspring, resulting in children with mental attributes surpassing their physical ones.

Therefore, the education of a child should commence long before their arrival, with the mother's intentional cultivation of desired qualities through mental imagery and affirmation during pregnancy.

The child conceived in this manner will likely be receptive to positive suggestions, which can be transformed into beneficial autosuggestions that shape their life's trajectory. It's essential to understand that our words and actions are predominantly influenced by autosuggestions, often stemming from examples or verbal suggestions.

To guide children effectively, parents and educators must be mindful of avoiding the instigation of negative autosuggestions while fostering positive ones. When interacting with children, maintain a consistently calm demeanor and communicate in a gentle yet firm tone. This approach cultivates obedience without evoking any inclination to challenge authority.

Above all, it's crucial to refrain from harshness and brutality, as these behaviors risk instilling negative autosuggestions of cruelty and hatred. Instead, prioritize kindness and empathy to nurture a healthy psychological environment for the child's development.

Furthermore, it's crucial to refrain from speaking ill of others in the presence of children, as is often done when absent individuals are criticized casually. Such negative behavior sets a harmful example that children may mimic, potentially leading to disastrous consequences in the future.

Instead, foster in children a curiosity about the world and a love for nature by providing clear explanations and engaging them in cheerful discussions. Encourage their questions and address them pleasantly, avoiding dismissive responses like, "You're bothering me, be quiet, you'll learn that later."

Never resort to derogatory remarks like "You're lazy and good for nothing" when speaking to a child, as this can reinforce the very faults you accuse them of. It's essential to uplift and encourage children, guiding them towards positive behaviors and self-esteem.

When dealing with a child who exhibits laziness or performs tasks poorly, it's beneficial to provide positive reinforcement. Even if their work is not up to par, praise their efforts sincerely by saying something like, "This time, your work is much better than usual. Well done." This encouragement, though perhaps not entirely true at first, can boost the child's confidence and motivation. Over time, with consistent and judicious praise, the child will likely improve their work habits and become more diligent.

Additionally, it's essential to refrain from discussing illness in front of children, as this can instill negative autosuggestions in their minds. Instead, teach them that health is the natural state of being and that sickness is an anomaly that can be prevented by maintaining a balanced and regular lifestyle. By fostering a positive mindset around health and wellness, children can develop habits that contribute to their overall well-being.

Avoid instilling fear in children by teaching them to be afraid of various elements such as cold, heat, rain, or wind. Man is naturally equipped to withstand these variations without harm, and children should learn to adapt to them without complaint.

Furthermore, refrain from filling children's minds with stories of ghosts and monsters, as this may cultivate unnecessary fear and anxiety that could persist into adulthood. Instead, focus on fostering confidence and resilience in children.

When selecting caregivers or educators for children, it's essential to choose individuals who not only love them but also possess the qualities you wish to instill in your children. Surrounding them with positive role models can greatly influence their development.

Encourage a love of learning and work by presenting information in an engaging and pleasant manner. Provide clear explanations and incorporate anecdotes that spark curiosity and eagerness for the next lesson. By making learning enjoyable, you can inspire children to be enthusiastic and motivated in their studies and tasks.

Above all, instill in children the importance of work for human fulfillment, emphasizing that those who do not engage in productive activities lead unfulfilled lives. Work not only brings a sense of satisfaction but also prevents idleness, which can lead to various negative consequences such as weariness, neurasthenia, and even immoral behavior.

Teach children the values of politeness and kindness toward all individuals, regardless of their social status or age. Encourage them to show respect to those less fortunate and to refrain from mocking or belittling others for their physical or moral shortcomings.

Promote a sense of empathy and compassion in children by teaching them to love all humanity without prejudice. Emphasize the importance of helping those in need and encourage them to prioritize the well-being of others over their own self-interest. By fostering a sense of altruism and generosity, children can contribute positively to society and cultivate meaningful relationships with others.

Instill in children a sense of self-confidence by nurturing their belief in their abilities and potential. Teach them to approach challenges with rationality and thoughtfulness, rather than impulsiveness, by carefully considering all factors before making decisions. Encourage them to trust their reasoning and judgment, while also remaining open to new information that may alter their perspective.

Above all, emphasize the importance of having a clear and unwavering belief in one's ability to succeed in life. Teach children that success is not a matter of mere chance, but rather the result of deliberate effort and determination. Encourage them to actively pursue their goals with dedication and perseverance, knowing that their belief in their own success will propel them forward and guide their actions towards achieving their aspirations.

Parents and educators must lead by example, demonstrating in their own lives the principles they wish to instill in children. Children are highly impressionable and observant, often imitating the behaviors and attitudes of those around them. Therefore, it is essential for adults to embody the qualities of self-confidence, perseverance, and belief in success that they seek to cultivate in children.

When children witness adults who confidently pursue their goals, seize opportunities, and overcome challenges with determination, they are more likely to internalize these values and apply them in their own lives. Conversely, if adults display self-doubt, hesitation, or a lack of initiative, children may adopt similar attitudes and struggle to fulfill their potential.

By setting a positive example and demonstrating the power of self-belief and proactive action, parents and educators can inspire children to embrace opportunities, overcome obstacles, and ultimately achieve success in their endeavors.

Repeating affirmations such as **"Day by day, in all ways, I grow better"** can indeed be a powerful tool for instilling positive beliefs and attitudes in children. Consistently reinforcing these affirmations can help shape their mindset and contribute to their overall well-being.

Additionally, offering suggestions to children while they sleep, as described, can potentially influence their subconscious mind and promote the development of desired qualities and behaviors. This technique, known as bedtime suggestion or hypnopaedia, aims to leverage the suggestibility of the mind during sleep to reinforce positive messages and facilitate personal growth.

However, it's essential to approach these practices with caution and mindfulness. Parents and caregivers should prioritize the child's autonomy and consent, ensuring that the affirmations and suggestions align with the child's values and goals. Additionally, it's crucial to maintain a supportive and nurturing environment where children feel empowered to express themselves and pursue their aspirations freely.

Overall, incorporating positive affirmations and bedtime suggestions into a child's routine can be a valuable complement to their upbringing, fostering resilience, self-confidence, and a positive outlook on life.

By guiding students through affirmations and encouraging them to adopt positive attitudes and behaviors, teachers can help cultivate a mindset conducive to personal growth and academic success.

The suggested morning routine for teachers to lead students in affirmations is a thoughtful approach to instilling values such as kindness, obedience, and appreciation for learning. By prompting students to reflect on the importance of these qualities and their intrinsic value, teachers can help them develop a sense of responsibility and empathy towards others.

Furthermore, encouraging students to approach their lessons with enthusiasm and openness to learning can foster a love for knowledge and intellectual curiosity. By framing learning experiences as opportunities for growth and discovery, teachers can inspire students to engage actively in their education and embrace challenges with confidence.

It's important for teachers to tailor their approach to the individual needs and developmental stages of their students, ensuring that affirmations are delivered in a manner that resonates with each student's unique personality and learning style. By incorporating positive suggestions into their daily routines, teachers can play a significant role in nurturing students' social-emotional development and academic achievement.

Emile Coué's counsel emphasizes the importance of focus, diligence, and self-discipline in the pursuit of academic success and personal development. By encouraging students to prioritize their attention during lessons, refrain from distractions, and remain dedicated to their studies, Coué aims to empower them with the tools they need to excel academically and cultivate strong character traits.

The affirmation that **"you are all intelligent"** serves to instill confidence and self-belief in students, fostering a positive mindset that is essential for overcoming challenges and achieving goals. By affirming their inherent intelligence, students approach learning with optimism and enthusiasm, recognizing their potential for growth and success.

Moreover, the importance of concentration and focus in the learning process. By teaching students to devote their full attention to their studies and tasks at hand, he equips them with essential skills for effective learning and retention of knowledge. Coué's emphasis on the importance of concentration highlights the role of mindfulness and presence in academic achievement and personal development.

Overall, Coué's counsel serves as a valuable reminder of the power of positive thinking, self-discipline, and focused effort in achieving success in both academic and personal endeavors. By internalizing these principles and incorporating them into their daily lives, students can cultivate the qualities necessary for realizing their full potential and leading fulfilling lives.

"ALL THAT WE THINK BECOMES TRUE FOR US. THEREFORE, WE MUST NOT THEN ALLOW OURSELVES TO THINK WRONGLY."

This statement emphasizes the profound influence of our thoughts on our reality. It underscores the importance of maintaining positive and constructive thinking patterns to shape our experiences and outcomes in life. By being mindful of our thoughts and striving to think positively and truthfully, we can cultivate a more fulfilling and harmonious existence.

Think "My Trouble Is Going Away," Just as You Think You Cannot Open Your Hands.

The more you say: *"I will not,"* the more surely the contrary comes about. You must say: *"It's going away,"* and think it. Close your hand and think properly: *"Now I cannot open it."* Try! (she cannot), you see that your will is not much good to you.

Observation.--This is the essential point of the method. In order to make auto-suggestions, you must eliminate the will completely and only address yourself to the imagination, so as to avoid a conflict between them in which the will would be vanquished.

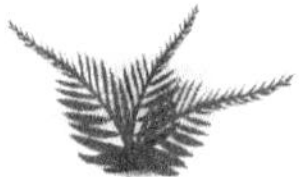

To become stronger as one becomes older seems paradoxical, but it is true.

These statements highlight the importance of adopting a positive mindset and utilizing the power of imagination in auto-suggestion. By focusing on the belief that one's troubles are diminishing or that positive changes are occurring, individuals can harness the subconscious mind to manifest desired outcomes. Additionally, the observations underscore the potential for improvement and healing, even in cases like diabetes, while also acknowledging the distinction between mere willpower and genuine desire for change.

After instructing them to close their eyes, M. Coué delivered a brief suggestive talk to his patients, similar to the one outlined in "Self

Mastery." Following this, he individually addressesed each patient, providing personalized encouragement tailored to their specific condition:

Addressing the first patient, he said, "You're experiencing pain, but I assure you that starting today, your unconscious mind will work to eliminate the root cause of this pain, whether it's arthritis or another issue. As the cause diminishes, so too will your pain, until it becomes insignificant in no time."

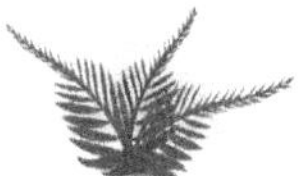

To the second person, M. Coué said, "Your stomach is experiencing dysfunction, possibly with some dilation. However, as I mentioned earlier, your digestive system will progressively improve. Furthermore, the dilation of your stomach will gradually diminish. Your body will restore the strength and elasticity your stomach has lost, allowing it to regain its original shape and perform its functions more efficiently. As this occurs, any pouch formed by the relaxed stomach will shrink, preventing food from stagnating and reducing fermentation until it disappears completely."

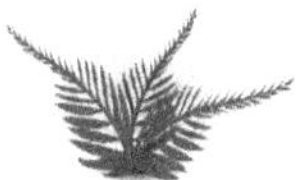

To the third person, M. Coué assures, "Regardless of any liver lesions you may have, your body is actively working to heal them every day. As these lesions gradually disappear, the symptoms you're experiencing will diminish and eventually fade away. Your liver will function more normally, producing alkaline bile in the right quantity and quality, which will aid in intestinal digestion."

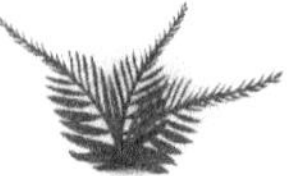

Addressing the fourth person, he advises, "Listen closely, my child. Whenever you feel an attack coming on, remember my words: 'No, no! You will not have that attack, and it will fade away before it even begins.'"

He continues this personalized approach for each individual, providing tailored suggestions based on their specific conditions and needs.

After attending to each individual, M. Coué instructs everyone to open their eyes and states, *"You have heard the advice I've just given you. To put it into practice, here's what you must do: Every morning before getting out of bed, and every evening before going to sleep, close your eyes to focus your attention. Repeat the following phrase twenty times, moving your lips (this is essential) and counting mechanically on a string with twenty knots: 'Every day, in every way, I am getting better and better.'"*

It's important not to focus on any specific aspect, as the phrase *"in every way"* encompasses all aspects of improvement. This autosuggestion should be made with confidence, faith, and the certainty of achieving the desired outcome. The stronger the person's conviction, the greater and more rapid the results will be.

Additionally, whenever you experience any physical or mental discomfort throughout the day or night, affirm to yourself that you will not consciously contribute to it and that you will make it disappear. Then, try to isolate yourself as much as possible. If it's a mental discomfort, pass your hand over your forehead; if it's physical, focus on the painful area. Repeat quickly, moving your lips, the words: ***"It is going, it is going..."* for as long as necessary.** With practice, you'll find that the discomfort disappears in about 20 to 25 seconds. Repeat this process whenever necessary.

For this, as for other autosuggestions, it's crucial to act with confidence, conviction, and faith, and most importantly, without effort.

M. Coué also emphasizes the importance of being aware of our thoughts and avoiding negative autosuggestions. If we slip up, we should hold ourselves accountable and acknowledge our mistake.

As a grateful admirer of M. Coué's work, I must say that he brilliantly demonstrates that the power to achieve health and happiness lies within us. By eliminating self-inflicted suffering and embracing self-awareness, as advised by Socrates and Pope, we can fully harness the benefits of autosuggestion.

Extracts from Letters Addressed to M. Coué

Dear M. Coué,

I am thrilled to share with you the news of my success in the English secondary Certificate examination. Just two hours ago, the final results were posted, and I am delighted to inform you of my achievement, particularly in relation to my performance during the viva voce examination. I passed with flying colors and experienced minimal nervousness, which used to plague me with intolerable nausea before tests. Remarkably, I maintained a sense of calm throughout the examination, impressing the jury with my apparent self-possession.

To my surprise, the tests I once dreaded the most turned out to be the ones where I excelled the most. The jury honored me with a Second place, and I attribute much of my success to the assistance you provided. Your guidance undoubtedly gave me an advantage over the other candidates.

Thank you once again for your invaluable help.

Warm regards,

Mlle. V----

Schoolmistress, August 1916

Dear M. Coué,

I am writing to express my heartfelt gratitude for the tremendous benefit I have gained from your method. Prior to seeking your help, I struggled immensely to walk even 100 yards without becoming breathless. However, thanks to your guidance, I can now walk for miles without feeling fatigued. Remarkably, I am able to walk from rue du Bord-de-l'Eau to rue des Glacis, a distance of nearly four kilometers, several times a day and with ease.

Moreover, the asthma that once plagued me has almost completely disappeared.

Please accept my sincerest thanks for your assistance.

With gratitude,

Paul Chenot

Rue de Strasbourg, 141 Nancy, Aug. 1917

Dear M. Coué,

I am at a loss for words to express my gratitude to you. Thanks to your guidance, I can proudly say that I am almost completely cured, and I have been eagerly awaiting this moment to convey my heartfelt thanks.

I suffered from two varicose ulcers, one on each foot. The ulcer on my right foot, which was as large as my hand, has miraculously healed entirely. After weeks of being confined to bed, I received your letter, and almost immediately, the ulcer on my right foot healed, allowing me to get up and move around. While the ulcer on my left foot is not yet fully healed, I am confident that it will be soon.

I faithfully recite the prescribed formula every night and morning, and I have complete confidence in its effectiveness. Additionally, I must mention that my legs were as hard as stone, and I could not bear even the slightest touch. Now, I can press them without experiencing any pain, and I can walk once more, which brings me immense joy.

With deepest gratitude,

Mme. Ligny

Mailleroncourt-Charette (Haute Saône), May 1918

The Miracle Within

(Reprinted from the "Renaissance politique, littéraire et artistique" of the 18th of December, 1920)

HOMAGE TO EMILE COUÉ

In September 1920, I had the opportunity to delve into Charles Baudouin's book "Suggestion et Autosuggestion" for the first time. Authored by Baudouin, a professor at the Institute J. J. Rousseau in Geneva, Switzerland, the book is dedicated to Emile Coué with deep gratitude. Published by Delachaux and Niestle in Paris, the book captivated me from start to finish.

Baudouin's work presents a simple yet profoundly humanitarian approach founded on a theory that might seem simplistic precisely because it is accessible to all. However, its potential impact, if universally applied, is immense and far-reaching.

Emile Coué, who currently resides in Nancy, France, has dedicated more than twenty years of tireless effort to this cause. Coué, deeply influenced by the work and experiments of Liébault, the pioneer of the doctrine of suggestions, has focused his attention on promoting the cultivation of autosuggestion among his fellow human beings.

At the turn of the century, Emile Coué achieved the culmination of his research, unlocking the vast potential of autosuggestion. Through countless experiments involving thousands of subjects, he demonstrated the power of the unconscious mind in influencing organic conditions. This breakthrough was revolutionary, as it offered a remedy for afflictions previously deemed incurable or excruciatingly painful, offering hope where none existed before.

Though delving into the intricate scientific details is beyond the scope of this discussion, I will outline how the method practiced by the learned man from Nancy operates.

Embodying the essence of a lifetime dedicated to patient investigation and continuous observation, Coué's method is encapsulated in a concise formula to be repeated twice daily. This ritual entails speaking softly, with eyes closed and the body in a relaxed position, ideally while lying in bed or seated in a comfortable chair. The tone of voice should resemble that of reciting a litany, imparting a sense of reverence and conviction. The transformative mantra consists of the following words: "Every day, in every respect, I am getting better and better."

Coué's method entails repeating the phrase "Every day, in every respect, I am getting better and better" twenty times, facilitated by a rosary-like string with twenty knots, ensuring a mechanical recitation vital for its effectiveness. This physical detail holds significance, as it ensures the disciplined repetition necessary for the subconscious to register the message.

During this recitation, one should refrain from focusing on any particular ailment or worry; instead, they should adopt a passive state of mind, accompanied by the simple desire for improvement. The phrase "in every respect" carries a broad, encompassing effect, addressing various aspects of one's well-being.

Crucially, this expression of desire should be devoid of passion or willfulness, conveyed with gentleness yet absolute confidence. Coué emphasizes the exclusion of the will during autosuggestion; instead, it is the imagination—the potent force far more dynamic than conventional willpower—that must be invoked.

"Have confidence in yourself," advises Coué, encouraging unwavering belief in the positive outcomes envisioned. Indeed, those who possess faith, bolstered by persistence, find themselves on the path to wellness and self-improvement.

The testimony provided by Charles Baudouin's volume deeply impacted me. It detailed the cure of various ailments, including serious conditions like tuberculosis, which conventional medicine often struggles to treat effectively. One case, in particular, stood out—the recovery of a woman named Mme. D----, who had advanced tuberculosis yet was cured without relapse, even becoming a mother afterward. Such examples seemed nothing short of miraculous, especially considering the failure of conventional medical treatments.

This revelation came at a time when I was suffering from acute neuritis in my face for two years. Despite consulting four doctors, including specialists, they all offered the same grim prognosis: "Nothing to be done!" Hearing this repeatedly only exacerbated my suffering, as it reinforced a sense of hopelessness and despair.

Armed with the simple yet powerful formula provided by the Coué Method, I began reciting it with unwavering faith. Despite the rain and wind, I ventured into the garden, repeating the affirmations softly to myself: "I am going to be cured, I shall have no more neuritis, it is going away, it will not come back, etc." The next day, to my immense joy, I found myself cured of the abominable complaint that had made life unbearable for so long. The skeptics may attribute it to mere nervousness, and I concede that point to them gladly. But buoyed by this success, I decided to apply the Coué Method to other ailments.

Next, I targeted an oedema in my left ankle, a condition resulting from a kidney disorder deemed incurable by conventional medicine. Remarkably, within just two days of practicing the Coué Method, the oedema had vanished entirely. Encouraged by these results, I continued to apply the method to other issues, such as fatigue and mental depression, with extraordinary improvements.

Filled with gratitude and admiration for my newfound benefactor, I made the journey to Nancy to personally thank Emile Coué. There, I encountered a man of exceptional kindness and simplicity, who quickly became not only my benefactor but also my friend.

It was absolutely necessary for me to witness Emile Coué in action, to see the Coué Method applied firsthand. He graciously invited me to attend one of his popular "séances," where I witnessed an orchestra of gratitude. People with lung lesions, displaced organs, asthma, even Pott's disease, and paralysis, a myriad of seemingly incurable ailments, were experiencing remarkable improvements. I saw a paralytic, who had been contorted and immobile in their chair, miraculously rise and walk. Emile Coué's message was clear: have unwavering confidence in yourself, believe in your ability to heal, and your spirit will respond, bringing about physical and mental well-being.

Emile Coué never claimed to cure anyone himself; he merely showed individuals how to unlock the power within themselves to heal. He approached the paralytic and asked if they believed they could walk. With a resounding "Yes," the individual rose and walked, a true miracle unfolding before my eyes.

Another young girl, afflicted with Pott's disease, shared with me the intense joy of feeling herself come back to life after believing herself to be beyond hope. Three women, cured of lung lesions, expressed their gratitude at being able to return to work and lead normal lives once again.

In the midst of these miraculous transformations, Emile Coué stood out as a singular figure. He seemed to transcend the ordinary, driven not by monetary gain but by genuine love and compassion for those he helped. His work was entirely selfless, and he refused to accept any payment for it. When I expressed my profound gratitude to him, he simply replied, "No, I owe you nothing. My only satisfaction comes from seeing you continue to enjoy good health."

There is an irresistible charm to this humble philanthropist, Emile Coué. As we walked arm in arm around his kitchen garden, which he tends to diligently each morning, I couldn't help but feel drawn to his simplicity and warmth. Emile Coué, almost a vegetarian, takes pride in the results of his labor in the garden.

Our conversation turned serious as he shared his profound insights: "Within your mind lies an unlimited power. It can influence matter if we know how to harness it. The imagination, like an untamed horse, can lead us astray if not directed properly. But with skillful guidance, it can take us wherever we desire. Autosuggestion, spoken aloud, is a command received by the unconscious, which then carries it out, often most effectively during sleep. Therefore, evening autosuggestion is of utmost importance and can yield marvelous results."

Emile Coué explained a simple technique for alleviating physical pain or mental distress: repeating the phrase "It is going away..." in a monotone voice while placing a hand on the affected area or on the forehead. This method, he assured me, is highly effective in soothing both mind and body.

Having experienced firsthand the profound impact of autosuggestion on my life, I urge you to embark on this journey yourself. I recommend starting with Charles Baudouin's book, followed by his pamphlet "Cultivating Moral Strength," and finally, Emile Coué's concise treatise "Self-Mastery." These resources can be obtained directly from Emile Coué in Nancy.

If, like me, you undertake this pilgrimage, you will come to admire this remarkable man and his boundless charity and love for humanity, echoing the teachings of Christ. And like me, you will find physical and mental healing, making life richer and more beautiful. Surely, this endeavor is worth pursuing.

With warm regards, M. Burnat-Provins

Some Notes on the Journey of M. Coué to Paris in October, 1919

Here are some notes on the journey of M. Coué to Paris in October 1919:

Desiring to ensure that the teachings of M. Coué during his visit to Paris in October 1919 are not lost to others, I have taken the initiative to document them. Setting aside the countless individuals who have experienced physical or mental healing through his benevolent treatment, let us focus on a few of his teachings:

Question: Why do I not achieve better results despite using your method and prayer?

Answer: It is likely because, deep down, there exists an unconscious doubt, or because you exert effort. Remember, efforts are driven by the will; if you engage the will, you risk activating the imagination in the opposite direction, thereby bringing about the opposite of what you desire.

Question: What should we do when something troubles us?

Answer: When faced with something troubling, immediately repeat to yourself, "No, that does not trouble me at all, not in the least. In fact, the situation is rather agreeable than otherwise." In essence, the idea is to channel our thoughts positively rather than negatively.

These teachings emphasize the importance of maintaining a positive mindset and avoiding the activation of the imagination in a negative direction. By consciously redirecting our thoughts and beliefs, we can cultivate a more positive outlook and potentially overcome various challenges and difficulties in life.

Question: Are the preliminary experiments necessary, even if they seem beneath the dignity of the subject?

Answer: No, they are not strictly necessary, but they are highly beneficial. Despite appearing trivial to some, these experiments serve to demonstrate three important principles:

> Every idea we hold in our minds becomes a reality for us and tends to manifest itself in our actions.
>
> When there is a conflict between the imagination and the will, the imagination invariably triumphs. Consequently, we end up doing the opposite of what we consciously desire.
>
> It is remarkably easy for us to implant any idea into our minds, as evidenced by our ability to effortlessly transition from thinking "I cannot" to "I can."

These experiments underscore the power of our thoughts and the influence they exert over our actions and behaviors. While they may seem simple, their implications are profound and can significantly impact our lives.

Question: Should the preliminary experiments be practiced at home?

Answer: No, it is not advisable to perform the preliminary experiments alone at home. Doing so may lead to failure due to difficulty in achieving the appropriate physical and mental state, which can undermine one's confidence.

Question: How should one handle thoughts of pain or trouble?

Answer: When experiencing pain or trouble, it is important not to avoid thinking about it. Instead, confront it directly by affirming, "I am not afraid of you." Just as facing a barking dog with confidence prevents it from attacking, facing challenges with courage diminishes their power over us.

Question: What should one do if faced with a setback?

Answer: If faced with a setback, retreat temporarily, but maintain the resolve to continue forward.

Question: How can we manifest our desires?

Answer: By repeatedly affirming what we desire, such as "I am gaining confidence," or "My memory is improving," we gradually realize these desires. Conversely, if we persistently affirm the opposite, it is the contrary outcome that will manifest. Our words have a profound influence on our reality, and what we consistently affirm quickly becomes reality within reason.

How to Practice Conscious Autosuggestion

Extract from Émile Coué's *"Self-Mastery through Conscious Autosuggestion"* (1922)

In his renowned work on self-mastery, Émile Coué lays out a simple yet powerful method for harnessing the mind's potential through conscious autosuggestion. He advises incorporating this practice into your daily routine, both in the morning upon waking and in the evening before retiring to bed.

Begin by closing your eyes and taking three deep breaths. Then repeating a specific phrase twenty times in succession, ensuring that you move your lips with each repetition. The chosen phrase, "Day by day, in every way, I am getting better and better," serves as a universal affirmation encompassing all aspects of improvement. It is essential to approach this exercise with unwavering confidence and faith, believing wholeheartedly in the positive outcomes it will bring. The stronger your conviction, the more profound and rapid the results will be.

Additionally, whenever you encounter physical or mental distress throughout the day or night, Coué advises taking immediate action. Affirm to yourself that you will not contribute to the distress consciously and that you will make it disappear. Find a moment of solitude, close your eyes, and gently pass your hand over your forehead for mental distress or the affected area for physical discomfort. Then, rapidly repeat aloud, moving your lips: "It is going, it is going," and continue for as long as necessary. With practice, you will witness the distress dissipating within a

mere 20 to 25 seconds. Repeat this process whenever needed, always mindful to avoid exerting unnecessary effort.

Coué's method offers a straightforward yet profound approach to self-mastery, empowering individuals to tap into the innate potential of their minds and achieve remarkable personal growth.

Closing Words

Emile Coué unveils the profound concept of autosuggestion, dispelling historical misinterpretations and underestimations. Despite its seemingly contemporary relevance, Coué asserts that autosuggestion's roots stretch back to the dawn of human civilization.

According to Coué, autosuggestion is an inherent ability embedded within every individual since birth, possessing a remarkable power to shape outcomes positively or negatively depending on its application. Recognizing and harnessing this power is not just advantageous but imperative, especially for professionals like psychologist, doctors, judges, lawyers, and educators.

Through conscious engagement with autosuggestion, individuals can prevent the inadvertent spread of harmful suggestions, potentially averting catastrophes, while implanting positive suggestions to foster physical wellness and emotional resilience. Coué proposes that by actively embracing autosuggestion, individuals can chart their own paths and guide others toward positive transformations and personal growth.

In mastering oneself through mindful self-suggestion, we unlock the potential for profound personal growth and positive impact on the world. Coué's work serves as a beacon in this journey, reminding us of the ancient wisdom inherent within each of us, waiting to be tapped into and harnessed for the greater good.

References:

Banerjee, S., Srivastav, A., & Palan, B. M. (1993). Hypnosis and self-hypnosis in the management of nocturnal enuresis: a comparative study with imipramine therapy. *American Journal of Clinical Hypnosis, 36*(2), 113-119.

Coué, E. (2018). Self mastery through conscious autosuggestion. In *Revival: Self Mastery Through Conscious Autosuggestion (1922)* (pp. 5-35). Routledge.

Druetta, R., & Falbo, C. (2014). *Docteurs et Recherche... Une aventure qui continue (Cahiers de recherche de l'École Doctorale en Linguistique Française n. 8)* (Vol. 8, pp. 1-250). EUT Edizioni Università di Trieste.

Fromm, E., Brown, D. P., Hurt, S. W., Oberlander, J. Z., Boxer, A. M., & Pfeifer, G. (1981). The phenomena and characteristics of self-hypnosis. *International Journal of Clinical and Experimental Hypnosis, 29*(3), 189-246.

Fromm, E., Brown, D. P., Hurt, S. W., Oberlander, J. Z., Boxer, A. M., & Pfeifer, G. (1981). The phenomena and characteristics of self-hypnosis. *International Journal of Clinical and Experimental Hypnosis, 29*(3), 189-246.

Fromm, E., Lombard, L., Skinner, S. H., & Kahn, S. (1988). The modes of the ego in self-hypnosis. *Imagination, Cognition and Personality, 7*(4), 335-349.

O'Neill, L. M., Barnier, A. J., & McConkey, K. (1999). Treating anxiety with self-hypnosis and relaxation. *Contemporary Hypnosis, 16*(2), 68-80.

Sacerdote, P. (1981). Teaching self-hypnosis to adults. *International Journal of Clinical and Experimental Hypnosis, 29*(3), 282-299.

Appendix

LA MAÎTRISE DE SOI-MÊME
Par L'Autosuggestion Consciente

Quatrième Partie

JE vous ai donné de bons conseils. . . . . J'ai fait ma part; c'est à vous maintenant de faire la vôtre: et c'est la plus importante.

Aussi longtemps que vous vivrez, aussi longtemps que vous vivrez, vous m'entendez bien, tous les matins, avant de vous lever, tous les soirs, dès que vous serez au lit, fermez les yeux et répétez vingt fois de suite, avec vos lèvres, assez haut pour entendre vos propres paroles, sans chercher à penser à ce que vous dites—si vous y pensez, c'est bien; si vous n'y pensez pas, c'est encore bien—et comptant machinalement sur une petite ficelle, munie de vingt noeuds, la phrase "Tous les jours, à tous points de vue, je vais de mieux en mieux." Il y a dans cette phrase cinq mots importants. Ce sont les mots *à tous points de vue*. Ils s'adressent à tout. Aux choses physiques aussi bien qu'aux choses morales. Il est donc tout à fait inutile de se faire des autosuggestions particulières, puisque chacune d'elles se trouve comprise dans les mots "à tous points de vue." Mais, ce que je vous recommande particulièrement, c'est de faire cette autosuggestion d'une façon toute simple, toute enfantine, toute machinale et surtout sans effort. Comme cela: "Tous les jours, *à tous points de vue*, je vais de mieux en mieux." "Tous les jours, *à tous points de vue*, je vais de mieux en

vais de mieux en mieux." "Tous les jours, *à tous points de vue*, je vais de mieux en mieux," etc. Comme si l'on récitait les litanies. Par la répétition, vous faites pénétrer mécaniquement dans votre inconscient, par l'oreille, la phrase qui est une idée "tous les jours, à tous points de vue, je vais de mieux en mieux."

Vous avez vu par les exemples, que je vous ai donnés, que, lorsque nous avons une idée dans l'esprit, cette idée devient une réalité dans le domaine de la possibilité. Donc, si vous vous mettez bien dans l'esprit l'idée "Tous les jours, à tous points de vue, je vais de mieux en mieux," tous les jours, à tous points de vue, vous allez de mieux en mieux.

De plus, comme je l'ai déjà dit, chaque fois que dans le courant de la journée ou de la nuit, vous éprouvez un mal physique ou moral, affirmez-vous à vous-même que vous allez le faire disparaître; alors, isolez-vous autant que possible, fermez les yeux, et vous passant la main sur le front, pour un mal moral, sur la partie douloureuse, pour une douleur physique, répétez, extrêmement vite, avec vos lèvres, les mots "ça passe, ça passe, etc," aussi longtemps que cela est nécessaire. Avec un peu d'habitude, la douleur physique ou morale disparaît au bout de quelques secondes. Recommencez aussi souvent qu'il le faudra.

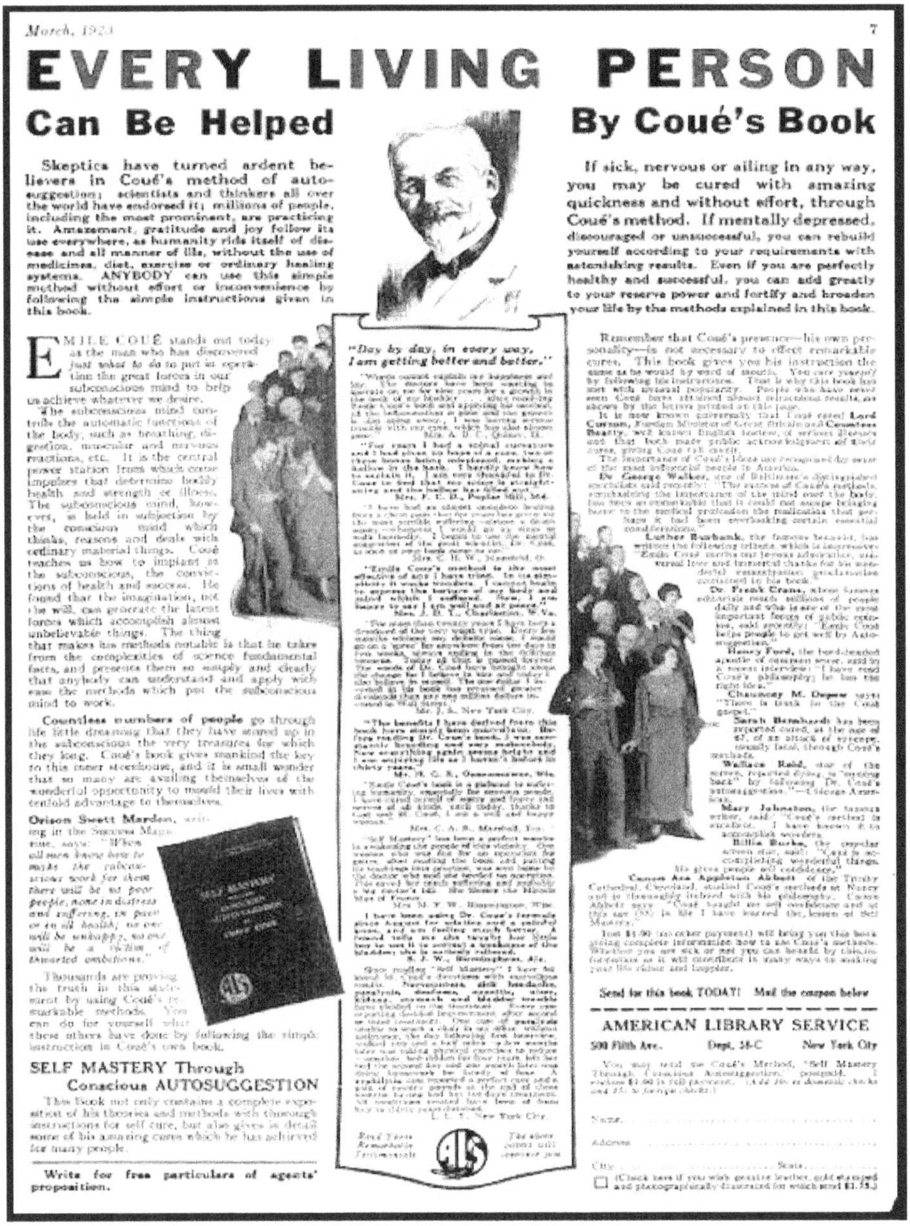

EVERY LIVING PERSON

Can Be Helped

By Coué's Book

Skeptics have turned ardent believers in Coué's method of auto-suggestion; scientists and thinkers all over the world have endorsed it; millions of people, including the most prominent, are practicing it. Amazement, gratitude and joy follow its use everywhere, as humanity rids itself of disease and all manner of ills, without the use of medicines, diet, exercise or ordinary healing systems. ANYBODY can use this simple method without effort or inconvenience by following the simple instructions given in this book.

EMILE COUÉ stands out today as the man who has discovered just what to do to put in operation this great forces in our subconscious mind to help us achieve whatever we desire.

The subconscious mind controls the automatic functions of the body, such as breathing, digestion, muscular and nervous reactions, etc. It is the central power station from which come impulses that determine bodily health and strength or illness. The subconscious mind, however, is held in subjection by the conscious mind which thinks, reasons and deals with ordinary material things. Coué teaches us how to implant in the subconscious, the convictions of health and success. He found that the imagination, not the will, can generate the latent forces which accomplish almost unbelievable things. The thing that makes his methods notable is that he takes from the complexities of science fundamental facts, and presents them so simply and clearly that anybody can understand and apply with ease the methods which put the subconscious mind to work.

Countless numbers of people go through life little dreaming that they have stored up in the subconscious the very treasures for which they long. Coué's book gives mankind the key to this inner storehouse, and it is small wonder that so many are availing themselves of the wonderful opportunity to mould their lives with tenfold advantage to themselves.

Orison Swett Marden, writing in the Success Magazine, says: "When all men knew how to make the subconscious work for them there will be no poor people, none in distress and suffering, in pain or in ill health; no one will be unhappy, no one will be a victim of thwarted ambitions."

Thousands are proving the truth in this statement by using Coué's remarkable methods. You can do for yourself what these others have done by following the simple instruction in Coué's own book.

SELF MASTERY Through Conscious AUTOSUGGESTION

This book not only contains a complete exposition of his theories and methods with thorough instructions for self cure, but also gives in detail some of his amazing cures which he has achieved for many people.

Write for free particulars of agents' proposition.

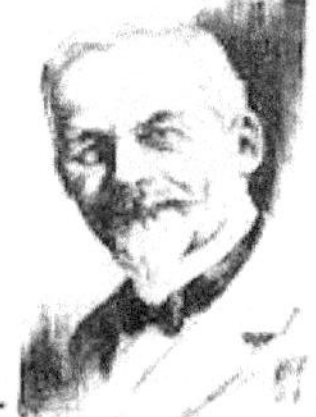

"*Day by day, in every way, I am getting better and better.*"

If sick, nervous or ailing in any way, you may be cured with amazing quickness and without effort, through Coué's method. If mentally depressed, discouraged or unsuccessful, you can rebuild yourself according to your requirements with astonishing results. Even if you are perfectly healthy and successful, you can add greatly to your reserve power and fortify and broaden your life by the methods explained in this book.

Remember that Coué's presence—his own personality—is not necessary to effect remarkable cures. This book gives you his instruction the same as he would by word of mouth. You cure yourself by following his instructions. That is why this book has met with universal popularity. People who have never seen Coué have attained almost miraculous results, as shown by the letters printed on this page.

It is now known universally that Coué cured **Lord Curzon**, Foreign Minister of Great Britain and **Countess Beatty**, well known English hostess, of serious illness and that both made public acknowledgment of their cures, giving Coué full credit.

The importance of Coué's ideas are recognized by some of the most influential people in America.

Dr. George Walker, one of Baltimore's distinguished specialists said recently: "The system of Coué's methods, emphasizing the importance of the mind over the body, has been so remarkable that it could not escape bringing home to the medical profession the realization that perhaps it had been overlooking certain essential considerations."

Luther Burbank, the famous botanist, has written the following tribute, which is impressive: "Emile Coué merits our fervent admiration, universal love and immortal thanks for his wonderful emancipation proclamation contained in his book."

Dr. Frank Crane, whose famous editorials reach millions of people daily and who is one of the most important forces of public opinion, said recently: "Emile Coué helps people to get well by Autosuggestion."

Henry Ford, the hard-headed apostle of common sense, said in a recent interview: "I have read Coué's philosophy; he has the right idea."

Chauncey M. Depew says: "There is much in the Coué gospel."

Sarah Bernhardt has been reported cured, at the age of 67, of an attack of syncope, usually fatal, through Coué's methods.

Wallace Reid, star of the screen, reported dying, is "coming back" by following Dr. Coué's autosuggestion.—Chicago American.

Mary Johnston, the famous author, said: "Coué's method is sunshine. I have known it to accomplish wonders."

Billie Burke, the popular screen star, said: "Coué is accomplishing wonderful things. He gives people self confidence."

Canon Asa Appleton Abbott, of the Trinity Cathedral, Cleveland, studied Coué's methods at Nancy and is thoroughly imbued with his philosophy. Canon Abbott says: "Coué taught me self confidence and at this age [50] in life I have learned the lesson of Self Mastery."

Just $1.90 (no other payment) will bring you this book giving complete information how to use Coué's methods. Whether you are sick or not you can benefit by this information it will contribute in many ways to making your life richer and happier.

Send for this book TODAY! Mail the coupon below.

AMERICAN LIBRARY SERVICE

500 Fifth Ave.   Dept. 3S-C   New York City

You may send me Coué's Method, "Self Mastery Through Conscious Autosuggestion," postpaid. I enclose $1.90 (a full payment). (Add 10c to domestic checks and 25c to foreign checks.)

Name ....

Address ....

City .... State ....

☐ (Check here if you wish genuine leather, gold stamped and stenographically decorated for which send $1.75.)

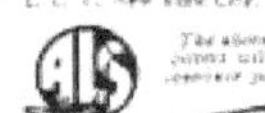

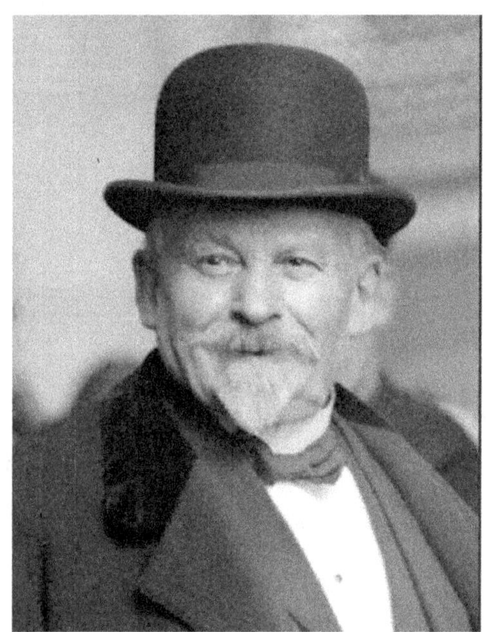

EMILE COUÉ